The
Shifted

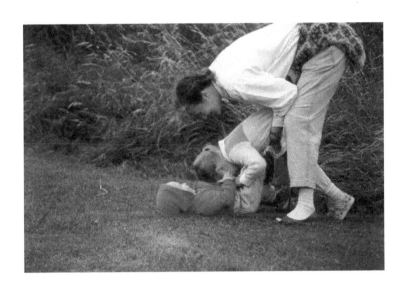

Michael
Goodell

White Bird Publications
P. O. Box 90145
Austin, Texas 78740
www.whitebirdpublications.com

ISBN: 978-1-63363-292-9
LCCN: 2018935635

PRINTED IN THE UNITED STATES OF AMERICA

This book is dedicated to Laura, Kate, Margaret, Becky, Martha, Jim, Lincoln, Mary Beth, James, Izzy and so many more than space allows me to mention. Your love and support made Mary's years so vital. Thank You.

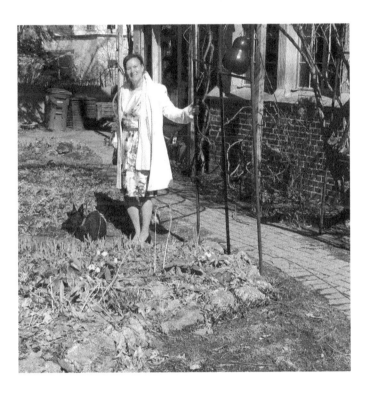

*Other Books by
Michael Goodell*

*Zenith Rising
Rebound*

The World Shifted

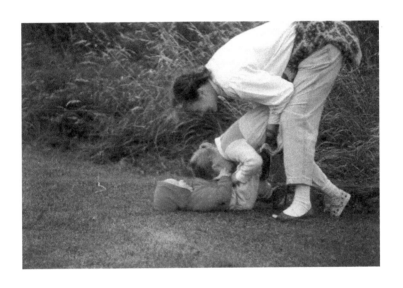

**White Bird
Publications**

March 16, 2010
The World Shifted

I'm sitting here surrounded by people sprawled enthralled by the omnipresent television. I'm killing time in the waiting room while my wife undergoes a routine colonoscopy. Turns out my buddy Dan is the anesthesiologist. He comes out and says, "I just knocked out your wife," and we share a laugh. I ask him when he's moving in, because he just bought a house around the corner. "Next week," he says.

"No loud parties," I joke. "I will call the cops. And tell your kids to stay off my land."

He laughs and says "I already told them, 'Remember the guy in Gran Torino?'"

He leaves, laughing. I leave in search of the cafeteria where I drink tepid coffee and eat a stale bran muffin, thinking how glad I am how little time I have to spend in places like this. Then I go back to the waiting room and discover the world has shifted on its axis.

They call my name. I go in. The doctor is there with color photos of all those places we're not meant to go. "It's cancer," he says, abruptly and emphatically. I go back to the waiting room and read the same paragraph twenty times and find it interesting how the magazine flutters in my hands. Dan comes out, claps me on the shoulder and tells me, "Anything you need, any time, call me."

She wakes up. I go in with the doctor. He barges straight in. I want to go first, hold her hand, but he's in the way. I hold her foot instead. He says it's cancer. She says, "Okay," blandly, as if he'd just told her she needed a haircut.

I think, "Whoa, where did that come from? It wasn't routine, and why am I the last to know?'

At home, she asks me to research rectal cancer online. It doesn't take long to learn that colorectal cancer is about the best kind of cancer to get, if you're going to get cancer. Very good survivability rates, depending on which stage you have. We agree she is probably Stage 1, maybe 2—3 at the worst.

Next comes a battery of tests. No way to study for them, and she flunks every one; our life is already in transition, the days a mad swirl. It's out of our control; we go where we're told to go and do what we're told to do. Monday Cat Scan. Wednesday pelvic sonogram. Before the latter, a visit to her primary care physician. She thinks it's to talk about the cancer. He thinks it's for a physical, which is why he's so surprised when I accompany her into the examining room. "No time for that," we say. "We need to get to the hospital for more tests." He brings up the Cat scan results, glances at us in dismay, and says, "No charge for this visit. Here, I'll give you copies of the report."

We read them at the hospital. It catches my eye, "Findings in keeping with rectal cancer and hepatic metastases." I'm not a doctor, nor do I play one on TV, but I don't like the sound of this.

She goes in for the procedure. I text a doctor friend. "Is this as bad as it sounds?" He texts right back, "Call me if you can."

The procedure over, I go in. The doctor comes. More bad news. Now things are really speeding up. We go home. I make her some soup. We sit in front of the computer again and look at our new, revised prospects. She keeps saying, "Well, it's Stage 3 then. Not as good as 2 or 1, but we can get through this." I know that's not right, but I don't argue. This is not an argument I want to win. She keeps looking, then she says, dully, "Oh, it's Stage 4."

We go back to the survival odds page, as if maybe, who knows, they refreshed it while we were gone, new results from outlying precincts or something.

But no, it's the same as before: Stage 4—only six percent survive Stage 4.

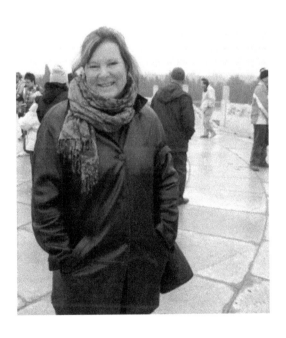

Photo by Emily Goodell

August 10, 2017
The First Time the World Shifted

On March 3, 2010, my wife, Mary Northcutt, went in for what was supposed to be a routine colonoscopy. They found cancer. We learned the cancer had metastasized to her lymph nodes and her liver. Our life, the life we had built and expected to continue to live, came screeching to a halt. We became exiles from that life. We emigrated to the horrible place known as Cancer Land.

Yet the story didn't start two years ago, but on another late winter afternoon nearly four decades before, in the cafeteria of a small Christian college in Southern California, when my friend, Tim Jones, looked out the window and remarked, "Oh, there's Mary."

I glanced up, thinking he meant Mary Wilson. The last person I expected to see was Mary Northcutt. She was supposed to be spending spring semester in England. But it was her, and when I saw her, I jumped up, raced through the crowded dining room, and sprinted around the perimeter of the building. When I reached her, I picked her up, and spun her round and round in my arms. By the time I set her down, her face flushed with amazement and surprise, I realized the world had shifted on its axis, and my life was never going to be the same.

I asked her to marry me on our first date. She said she was never going to get married. She moved to the mountains above Santa Cruz. When I moved to San Francisco, she moved to Michigan. I wrote her passionate love letters, which usually started out with a florid description of that day's sunset, as viewed from the roof of my apartment building. When I begged her to come to San Francisco, I felt like the hapless subject of a sappy Kenny Chesney song, though in no way did she want to be known as the Number One Fan of the Man from wherever I happened to be at the time.

It took some time, but I finally wore down her resistance. I had to follow her halfway across the country, but eventually, she agreed to marry me. We raised two children. We built a comfortable life with plenty of friends and a wealth of pleasures. Life was good, and there was no reason to expect it to change. Until that day five years ago when the world shifted again.

We were fortunate, in the early going, to have so many friends in the medical profession. One of them, a radiation oncologist, was tremendous. The first thing he did was explain exactly what was going to happen, every step of the way. What tests would be run, and why, and what we could expect. After each test, he told us what the results meant, and which options remained.

Paul, and several other friends, recommended doctors, surgeons, oncologists, all the best ones in their respective fields. We discovered that Metropolitan Detroit is blessed with a rich selection of top-notch Health Care Systems. We received services from three of them, and consulted with surgeons in four, and discovered there were still two or three major ones we never got around to.

Our friends' knowledge and advice were priceless, because we were babes in the woods. We had both been healthy our entire lives. We had no clue how hospitals worked, and what people did in them. We had never practiced or prepared for dealing with cancer. As dismaying and bewildering as it was, it would have been so much worse without our friends to point out the signposts.

Though I didn't set out to write a memoir about Mary's battle with cancer, I am a writer, and one way writers make sense of the world is by writing it down. I wrote "The World Shifted," the essay that begins this book, for just that purpose. I never shared it with anyone, but before long, after we let go of our secret, I started sending regular updates.

One of the first challenges one faces upon hearing the dread news is information management. Who should know about the diagnosis? It's absurd, of course, but that's the way it unfolds. It's as if you believe if no one knows, it must not be real.

Family, of course, must know, and your closest friends— that's one of the discoveries you make along the way—the people you want to tell might not be the people you would normally expect. They may not be the people you see every day, or the couple you go out to dinner with every couple of weeks. It might be an old roommate from another city on the opposite coast, or a best friend from college you haven't seen in fifteen years.

For Mary and me the information management phase ended abruptly. That first Sunday after the worst diagnosis, when the first doctor said there was no chance of surgery, that our strategy would be chemotherapy and hope for the best, we debated whether we wanted anyone at church to know. We decided we didn't. But that was before the closing hymn. Amazing Grace, that old standard from the Baptist churches of our childhoods in Tucson, Arizona and Lodi, California. Over the years we had transitioned to the Lutheran church, and the particular one we then called home had a tendency to end the service with the most ponderous, unmelodic, unsingable songs in the hymnal.

So it was a treat to sing that old standard, yet suddenly,

as it took us back to our youths, and in some strange way, even further back, to the distant past of just two weeks ago, before the diagnosis, back when the world still rotated on its axis, we lost the joy of singing.

We started off strong, but as the song wore on our voices became rougher, more hesitant, and by the time we reached the words, "When we've been there 10,000 years, bright shining as the sun," we both gave up singing altogether. I looked at Mary. Tears streamed as freely down her face as they did down mine. We shared a sad smile. Our bid to manage the information had failed. Everyone knew something was wrong, and soon they would know what. No use denying it any longer.

Once they know you've got cancer, people respond differently to you. Some walk around on tenterhooks. They speak softly, and slowly, as if a loud noise might shatter you. They mean well, but it's almost as if they're already in mourning. They're always there for you, but sometimes you're not sure you want them there, patting your hand and trying to put the best face on the matter.

Then there are those who run away. They act like they're afraid they might catch your cancer. Sometimes they apologized to me. They said they knew they were wrong, were weak, but they just couldn't bear it. I told them it was okay. They couldn't help it. It wasn't their fault. I knew this was true, because I had always been one of the cowards myself. I remember when I lost my first close friend to cancer. He succumbed the day after his thirty-ninth birthday.

I wasn't there for him the way I meant to be, the way I needed to be, until one day, about six months since the last time I'd seen him, I got a call from a friend who said, "If you want to see Tom one last time, you'd better get down to Harper Hospital today."

I went. When I walked into his room, he looked like a corpse already. His body had shrunken so much that his head seemed abnormally large. I started to say, reflexively, what I would have routinely said, which was, "How you doing,

Tom?" The words died in my throat. It was hard to imagine asking a more stupid question. Instead, I said—nothing. I just stood there. And Tom just lay there, staring at me through his impossibly large eyes. I was speechless and ashamed, and I felt he was saying through those giant blank eyes, "Is that all you got for me, buddy? Nothing? Really?"

Now, I knew cognitively, and it was confirmed by others who were with him until the very end, that Tom wasn't staring at me. Tom probably couldn't see, and hadn't recognized me. His indictment of my behavior was actually my indictment, but it was an indictment, and I was ashamed. I took it as long as I could, and then I fled, vowing to do better next time, to be a friend. The next time came and went, and so did I, in full flight from friendship and responsibility. So I understood when those we thought were our friends ran away. They were still our friends, and no doubt they hated themselves for their failure.

The third response was the best one. That was the friend who came over to go walking with Mary in the morning or to take her out to lunch. To go shopping or to a movie. To be cheerful, upbeat, to pretend there was nothing wrong. They were lying to us, and to themselves as well, and that was just fine. They were welcome lies; they allowed us the luxury of feeling normal. Ironically, despite being so facile in their deceptions, these were also the ones who could get as deathly serious as they needed to be. They were the ones with whom we could talk calmly, dispassionately, about mortality. Incidentally, until you've done that, you haven't really lived.

No matter how they responded, everyone, Mary's friends and mine, wanted news about Mary. I started composing updates, mainly to spare the feelings of the ones who ran away, because they always felt obligated to preface their inquiry with an apology. The first one was an essay as well as an update. It was so well received that I did the next one the same way. After a while I realized I couldn't just send an email saying Mary was fine, or about to face surgery, or was handling the latest course of chemo as well as she did the last one. I needed a vignette or anecdote, and I had to write a coherent essay tying the story to the update, and draw a conclusion, and then I had to cap it off with a clever or allusive title.

When I started circulating these updates among friends and family, and the strangers they began to reach, one of my goals was to demystify the experience for others. Not everyone is lucky enough to have so many friends in the medical profession to point the way. I wanted to let them know what we were up to, so if they ever had to face what we faced, perhaps they wouldn't have to go it alone.

This is a story about Mary's battle with cancer. It's a story of her courage, and her grace under pressure. Of her refusal to surrender to despair. She never stopped fighting. She was an inspiration to me, to her children, and to all her friends and hundreds of strangers who have shared her story. More than just a memoir about cancer, this is also a love story, a tale of heroism, and the restorative power of friends and family.

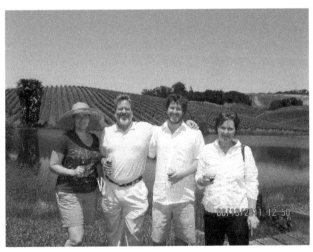

Mary enjoyed good wine, good food and good company in beautiful places, as captured in this photograph of daughter Emily, husband Michael, son Matthew, and Mary, on a 2008 trip to Napa Valley.

—Photo by Alan Phillips

April 9, 2010
The Other C-Word

Our first consultation wasn't very good. "No surgery," Dr. B. said, giving rise to that dread phrase, "inoperable cancer," and to our nickname for him, Dr. Doom. His game plan was chemotherapy and hope for the best. Mary asked about radiation. "Only for palliative purposes," he replied. Later, Mary said, with grim intensity, born of her experience taking care of her father as he died from a brain tumor, "I know what palliative means." It was as if he were sticking a knife into her, and by extension, into me.

That was Friday, March 14. That Sunday was when our information control strategy crashed and burned during the closing hymn. Now Mary's name is mentioned each week during Prayers for the People.

Our second consultation went better. Dr. R. wasn't ready to rule out surgery. If the chemo takes hold, we might have a chance at rectal surgery, and possibly liver surgery, too. This was much more appealing, so much so that I suggested we keep consulting with doctors until we find one who says she doesn't have cancer. And that's the one we'll go with.

During our third consultation the surgeon brought up the other C-word, as in, "If we hit this aggressively, and Mary responds, there is a chance that we can cure this." We definitely like the sound of that.

So this is our status as of today. Tomorrow Mary goes in for a minor surgical procedure, the installation of her mediport. Then next Monday we start chemotherapy. The treatments will last three days, and then Mary will rest until April 26th, when she will repeat the treatment. Our plan right now is to continue the two-week cycle of treatments for three or four months, and then repeat the various scans to see how the tumors have responded.

Our oncologist is optimistic. He says Mary has three things in her favor. She is relatively young, she is in good health, and she is not presenting any symptoms. This means we can hit it harder and longer than we could if circumstances were different. Mary is eager to get started. She says, "I want to get started, and I want to kill this thing."

Those who know Mary well know this is uncharacteristically harsh speech for her. In fact, I doubt she's ever used the word "kill," except, perhaps, from time to time in reference to me, when I came home a little later than promised, and at other times, also directed at me, as in "All right, I'll kill the spider, you big baby."

Our attitude is good. We are going into this planning to win. It is strange how, in the short course of four weeks one can go from blithe existence to calmly discussing with strangers such matters as personal mortality. Yet we can and do now. We have come to understand that this, too, is part of life. It is the start of an amazing adventure.

We appreciate all the warm wishes, the kind gestures, and the offers of support; we value your prayers. Don't be strangers, and don't be afraid to call or email, or offer a shoulder to cry on, or a back to lean on.

April 11, 2010
Timing is Everything

Last Sunday, the day before her first chemotherapy treatment, Mary invited about a dozen people for brunch. It was a beautiful day, much warmer than expected. The women were dressed in pastels, and we all sat outside, sipped mimosas, and enjoyed a perfect spring afternoon. It was an inspired, and wonderfully defiant, way to begin the process.

Then we began the next stage in our journey. The chemo center was a large room lined with comfortable chairs occupied by patients in varying stages of their fight with cancer. It was interesting to see the unity and support everyone gave each other, wishing the others good luck as each one finished his or her treatment and left. There was laughter, and good spirits, and even those who were suffering the most were inspired to maintain a positive outlook.

It had been five hours by the time the last treatment was finished, and Mary was fitted with her pump, which would continue pumping for the next 48 hours. Everyone calls this drug 5-FU, which suggests, if nothing else, cancer specialists have a bizarre sense of humor.

Mary felt fine after the treatment, and upon returning home, she announced she was hungry. She had put a pot roast and some vegetables in a slow cooker before we left, and it was ready when we returned. So we had a late lunch, and then she dropped in on an Herb Society of America board meeting. I was thinking things had gone about as well as they could have, for the first day.

Later, she felt a little tired, and she noted that her jaw was sore. She said she had to warm up her jaw before she chewed anything, even a cracker, and yes, her mouth was very sensitive to hot and cold. But there was no nausea or any other form of discomfort.

Then, around 9:00 p.m., Mary's mother's caretaker called from Tucson. Nancy had another stroke, she announced. It sounded pretty bad, though Mary did get to speak to her mother. They said provisional goodbyes, and Mary discovered another side effect. When her tear ducts are activated, it sends sharp pains through her sinus cavities and down her jawline. We called Becky, Mary's life-long friend, and a nurse, who lives in Tucson. She visited Nancy, and emailed me this morning that she has stabilized, and is in no worse shape than before.

Which is fortunate, as this is definitely not the right time for that sort of complication. Those of you who are praying might consider tossing in one for Mary's mother as well.

April 26, 2010
Cocktails at the Cancer Bar

One of Mary's first reactions to the chemotherapy lab was to say it was a cancer bar, and they were serving radioactive cocktails. It's hard to tell exactly what the ingredients are, but they don't seem to be bothering her very much. In fact, she responded so well, with just general tiredness and a couple days of feeling queasy last Thursday and Friday, that Mary was wondering if the treatments were actually working. She thinks if they aren't making her sick, they probably aren't killing cancer cells either. But we both acknowledge that there's probably a cumulative effect to the treatments, and over time she'll probably feel worse. And then, we are confident, she will feel better again.

All the same, last week, actually, starting Saturday the 17th, Mary was back to normal. She got a head start on gardening, and enjoyed a great visit from her old friend and former roommate, Lori. We're planning to go up to Glen Lake this Friday for a long weekend.

By the way, Mary's mother has stabilized. We're not sure now if she actually had a stroke or if it was just a reaction to a change in medications. The important thing is she is okay right now. Mary's fortunate to have kept strong friendships in Tucson, especially with Martha and Becky, who visited Nancy and were able to reassure Mary. Plus, our son, Matthew is there, attending the University of Arizona, and visits his grandmother regularly.

When I told Matthew about Mary's diagnosis, his first response was, "Well, I should probably cancel the internship." He was scheduled to do an educational/social work project in Thailand, which he was very much looking forward to. Cancelling it was the right thing to do, and I will be forever grateful that he expressed it as a decision rather than a question, as in, "Should I cancel?"

The chemo lab offers a wide spectrum of the cancer experience. Most people have a friend or family member with them, and many exude good humor and a fighting spirit. For others, some of whom are further along in their treatments, life has lost much of its gloss. Yesterday we were there for four hours, and saw the full range on display.

The most painful to witness are the repeat visitors, the ones to whom the nurses say, "Oh, Lois, I'm so sorry to see you back." There is no mystery for them, no way to convince themselves they are embarking on an amazing journey. They know what to expect, how they are going to suffer. It is sad. There isn't anything we, mere rookies, can really say to these veterans. We can't offer the encouragement we can to others, and we can't cling to their positive spirits, because they are nowhere on display. It almost feels wrong to be too cheerful ourselves, as if somehow we're mocking them.

There's not much really to tell, which in this case is a good thing, but I figured it can't hurt to keep you up to date. Keep those thoughts and prayers coming, and if you're in town, don't be a stranger. Lunch is always a good idea, especially in the weeks after chemo, or every other week starting May 3rd.

May 12, 2010
Catching Days

On her blog, "Catching Days," Cynthia Martin features a quote from Annie Dillard, "How we spend our days is, of course, how we spend our lives." This resonates in a number of ways. The main one is the fact that Mary and I are spending our days, hence our lives, in a radically different manner than we had ever contemplated, starting just a little over two months ago.

On another level, catching days perfectly sums up the way we look at life now. No matter how optimistic our oncologists and surgeons may sound regarding Mary's prospects, and no matter how superbly she is tolerating treatment now, no matter how guilt-inspiringly good she feels, Stage 4 cancer remains a serious, critical threat to her future, and at the very least, a life-transforming experience.

As a result, we look at each day differently. We practice "catching days." This practice is greatly facilitated by Mary's continuing good health, for which we remain grateful. She finished her third cycle of chemo today, and decided to take a nap while I made some soup for lunch, so she would be rested for an Herb Society meeting tonight. And so it goes.

We're heading back up north this weekend, and out to California the following one, to attend my niece Marina's wedding. It will be a good chance to see my family, and to spend quality time with our children, Matthew and Emily. (Emily was here last weekend, and made a nice quiche for Mother's Day). It's liberating to have this freedom of movement, which greatly helps us catch each day.

Finally, an anecdote from the chemo lab. Monday a new patient made an appearance. The nurse asked him about his mediport. A mediport, for those who don't know, is a small device surgically installed beneath the skin, usually on the upper chest, and connected by a catheter to a vein. It allows repeated needle insertions with far less discomfort to the patient. When the nurse asked, "Which side is your port on?" the old sailor replied, "The port side."

"Yes, but which side?" she asked.

"The port side," he repeated.

They went back and forth a couple more times, by which point most of the other patients, their companions, and the rest of the nursing staff were convulsed in laughter. The old sailor rose above his affliction to bring joy to everyone around him; he allowed us all to catch that day.

June 4, 2010
That's the Good News?

Yesterday we consulted with Dr. A. He is pleased that Mary's blood counts have held up so well after four cycles of chemotherapy. The side effects continue to be mild, and he explained the difference between the neuropathy Mary thought she had and the sensitivity to cold which was actually bothering her. They are two completely different things, and the sensitivity should go away when she completes chemotherapy. Also, we agreed that the reason she felt so slammed by the last cycle might have more to do with the fact that she kept busy even during the chemo days, visiting nurseries and helping to plant gardens at the War Memorial. We agreed she needs to give chemo the respect it requires, for as long as the cycles continue.

Then again, she may not be finished with chemo as quickly as we had expected. The doctor suggested we might want to stick with it longer than the original plan, especially if it appears to be working. As long as she can handle it, she should keep going.

When we left, I said it was great to get good news. Mary

wondered what that was, so I said being able to take chemo longer than planned. "That's the good news?" she responded. Actually, it is. It may make her feel lousy, but it isn't making her sick, and it's not wearing her down as much as it could be. The longer we can do it, the more likely it is to beat down the tumors, and the better chance she has to have surgery, and to have a good outcome from it.

Mary stopped by the lab to have some blood drawn, so we could get a CEA reading. CEA, or carcinoembryonic antigens, are molecules occurring in the blood which serve as markers for cancer, especially colorectal cancer. Normal CEA levels are around 2.5 for nonsmokers or 5.0 for smokers. Although testing for CEA hasn't proved to be a completely reliable method of cancer screening, it can give some indication of the effectiveness of a particular course of treatment.

When Mary started chemo, her CEA was 238. After her appointment today, we walked down to The Hill Restaurant to meet Dick and Susan, friends who had invited us out for lunch. When we returned home, there was a message from Jeanine the PA at Dr. A.'s office, calling to say she had "Good news" about Mary's lab tests. Naturally, Mary decided to forestall her nap long enough to make the call. The news? Her CEA count is down to 186, a twenty-two percent reduction.

So that's the good news. It doesn't mean she's out of the woods yet, but it is definitely pointing in the right direction. It makes us more inclined to use "The Other C-Word." It makes our plans to visit Charlie and Kelly in Australia next spring, or to move up north and open a winery, or even, come on, to finish reroofing the house, less of an act of denial, a show of the sort of bravado shown by the man who refuses a blindfold when facing a firing squad, and more of the kind of practical long-range planning in which normal couples engage. (A word of advice to others who share my abhorrence of flying, who might find themselves in my situation: consider waiting for that first CEA test before committing to a twenty-hour-long flight across the South Pacific).

The bottom line is, the chemo appears to be working, and Mary is tolerating it remarkably well. We find ourselves surrounded by loving friends, and we continue to make plans, for next week, next month, and next year.

I hope, once we lick this thing, that we will always remember the value of friends, and the importance of reaching out, constantly reaffirming and refreshing them. It's so easy in our day to day lives to give in to the convenient friend, the acquaintance in place, and to neglect the possibly more valuable friendship which, owing to geography or conflicting schedules, is harder to connect with. But there is nothing more valuable in life than spending time with the ones you love. Maybe that's why we have to go through this, so we can learn that lesson all over again.

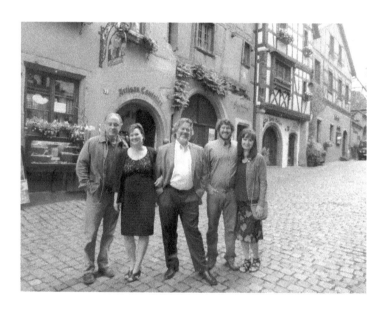

We celebrated our 30th anniversary in June, 2012 with friends and family in Alsace, France. From left, Nigel Adams, Mary, Michael, Matthew, Sabine Adams.
—Photo by Emily Goodell

June 28, 2010
No (Bad) News is Good News

Mary and Matthew walked to The Hill for a late lunch today. I met them there, after taking Emily to the airport. After lunch, we walked out to my car to discover a flat tire. We figured out where the jack and spare were located, and I jacked up the Escape. Matthew suggested it should be jacked higher, but I thought it was high enough. I took the tire off. He tried to put the other on. There wasn't enough clearance. Before either of us could act, Mary grabbed the jack and gave it a couple more cranks. So there Matthew and I were, standing around watching while Mary, in a pretty summer dress, sat on the ground jacking up the car. I told Matthew this was a pretty good look. He agreed it was a bit out of the ordinary.

"Don't worry," I assured him. "If anyone gives us a hard time, I'll just tell them she has cancer."

So the jokes just keep on coming. We had a good visit with Dr. A. today. Actually, all visits with Dr. A. were good. He was very upbeat, very caring, as if he had Mary's interests at heart. In other words, he fooled us for a very long time.

Still, at that appointment, we learned that everything is

still going in the right direction. Good numbers remain high, and bad numbers are going lower. It's been six cycles now, or twelve weeks. Mary said she's disappointed she hasn't lost any weight, though Dr. A. said that's a good thing. She recognizes the truth of that, but still, you're supposed to lose weight; that's the only benefit.

Matthew has been in town for three weeks and will be around for another one before going back to Arizona. Emily has been in and out, flying out to California for her viticulture research, and then today she flew to Europe for a tour of the Champagne, Alsace, and Mosel regions. She didn't want to go, but it was for school. I guess somebody has to do it.

Last week, Matthew and Emily both took Mary to chemo one day. It was a good experience for them, and for myself, I was surprised to learn how much it seemed like time off. There's a lesson. Even when it seems like there isn't any stress, the situation works on you from the inside. I wonder how I would be faring if things were more dire.

We've been spending as much time Up North as we can, between chemo weeks, and will be heading up on Wednesday for the Fourth. Bryan and Rachel will be joining us, and Matthew has a couple of friends coming up. Two weeks ago, James and Sophie came down from Montreal for three days, and we enjoyed dining and wining, along with Emily, throughout the Leelanau Peninsula.

We hope to see Charlie and Kelly Anne when they come in from Australia in a few days, and Mary's friend Martha is coming out for a visit later this month. Then in August, Malcolm and Caroline are coming over from England, and Mary Lou will fly in from Denver. We have such a busy schedule, it's hard to find time for being sick.

I took a header over my handlebars a month ago, badly bruising my ribs, and I think Mary enjoyed being the caregiver for a while. But now I'm back to normal, and still feeling my way through this process. It's tempting to take ownership of Mary's cancer, to be the public face and official cheerleader. Sometimes I think I carry it too far, not letting her make any decisions, and deciding for her how good she feels. Maybe it's better to lay back, and let her handle things more. Maybe it's better not to be such a Pollyanna. Maybe we're ignoring some negative developments in our enthusiasm to be responding so well to her treatments.

It's hard to tell sometimes, which is why it was good to have Matthew and Emily here, so I could ask them if they noticed any changes. You know how it is with infants. They develop steadily and relentlessly, but the parents often don't register it, because it is incremental. It is only someone who hasn't seen the child for a month or two who can see the growth. Fortunately, they didn't see any changes for the worse.

One thing I have noticed since the weather has turned warm, (or hellishly hot, depending on your perspective), is Mary's and my response to temperature. Always at great variance, it has grown even greater. Sometimes I will walk into the sunroom complaining about the heat, to find Mary snuggled under a blanket. This always makes us laugh.

Anyway, things are continuing to go about as well as they can. Mary continues to live a full life, and her spirits are good and her confidence high. We have another CT Scan scheduled in three weeks, which will tell us how far she's come, and what our options will be going forward. Please keep Mary in your thoughts and prayers, and as always, don't be a stranger.

July 7, 2010
The Gift of Needing

One of the hardest things I've had to learn since Mary's diagnosis is the importance of accepting offered help. Harder still is learning to ask. Having always fancied myself as self-reliant, I have on occasion in the past gone without rather than ask for a favor. Lately though, I've come to view self-reliance as a form of selfishness. By refusing to ask for help, I am denying others the opportunity to give, of themselves, their time, their interest. Their giving to Mary is a form of self-assurance, a way to feel better about themselves in relation to Mary, or to us; it gives others the sense of partnership, of sharing in our battle.

So it was Tuesday, after the long holiday weekend, that Rachel took Mary to chemo. I had a conflict. A small one, taking Matthew to the airport, but a conflict just the same. And Rachel got to help. She got to lend a hand, and Mary was the beneficiary of another's kindness.

I'll keep trying to take this lesson to heart as we continue on our journey. As for the journey itself, we sort of stubbed our toe today, when Mary got her latest CEA count. It had gone up slightly, from last month, though it's still down from the first one. Dr. A. says the numbers aren't entirely reliable, that he could take five different samples from the same person, and probably get five different counts. We'll go with that one. It makes sense, and it sounds good.

\#

However, next Tuesday, the 13th, Mary will take another test, a CT Scan, and it will be very important for her to pass that one. Unfortunately, there's no way to study for these kinds of tests, and there are no shortcuts.

So think of Mary, especially next Tuesday, and I hope to report some very good news in about a week.

July 14, 2010
Maybe That's Why She Never Cried

Back in the early days, which seem at once so long ago and so recent, when I was still weepy and sobbing, and snuffling things to Mary like, "If you're strong enough, you can help me get through this," she made an observation which I found perplexing at the time. "I wonder why I can't cry," she mused.

Maybe, just maybe, the reason she couldn't cry was there was nothing for her to cry about.

Yesterday Mary had her CT Scan. Afterwards, we had lunch at a place called Dockside Jack's, a ramshackle restaurant plunked down in the midst of a vast marina. It was overcast, and refreshingly cool, so we sat outside, beside the glass-smooth water. All around us, overgrown boats occupied their slips, and warehouses, cranes and gas docks littered the horizon. It was peaceful, simultaneously maritime and industrial. We had the place to ourselves, in contrast to the mighty pulsing nautical nightlife the establishment seemed designed to accommodate. I was trying to figure out the best way to find out what the test had revealed, though Mary seemed inclined to wait for our doctors' appointments in two weeks' time. This patient acquiescence in whatever the future holds is something that constantly amazes me.

That evening, however, she received a call from Dr. A., who had no compunction about waiting around to give her the news. Short of "There is no cancer," his news was about as good as it was possible to hear. The short version is that the chemo is working. The tumors in her liver have shrunk. As for the primary cancer, the report reads, "The rectal mass is no longer identified," which means that ugly tumor, the one of which Dr. Doom said, while flourishing the photo in my face four months ago, while Mary was coming up from the colonoscopy anesthesia, "It is cancer. I have no doubt. Even if the biopsy comes back negative, I can tell you, it's cancer," is not visible to the naked eye.

What this means is Mary will probably have surgery in a month or two. One of the worst things about cancer is that the prospect of undergoing a six-to-eight-hour operation is unalloyed good news. What this means is perhaps we have turned a corner. It is as Churchill said about another great conflict, "Now this is not the end. It is not even the beginning of the end. But it is, perhaps, the end of the beginning."

In other words, we aren't out of the woods just yet, but shafts of sunlight are beginning to slice through gaps in the canopy. Since a CT Scan doesn't work on a microscopic level, the absence of visual evidence doesn't mean the cancer is gone. In all likelihood, it isn't. But if it is no longer visible, it increases the chances that Mary can have surgery with no permanent damage. As for the liver tumors, we still don't know what that involves, but since Dr. Y. was reasonably optimistic about the prospects of success from a combination of surgery and Radiofrequency Ablation when they were larger and still growing, the fact that they have been reduced makes those prospects all the more appealing.

We have gone into this battle with the love and support of friends and families, and with ranks of self-described "Prayer Warriors" leading the charge. Thus far the forces for truth, justice, and the American Way are routing the forces of evil arrayed against us. We are reinforced by justifiable optimism as we approach the next phase.

Mary, being Mary, upon hearing the news from Dr. A., said, "No, congratulations to you." As for me, I'm seriously searching for a sedative to help me endure a twenty-hour flight to Australia next spring.

July 20, 2010
Both Ends of the Spectrum

Yesterday Mary started her eighth chemotherapy cycle. We don't know if it is her last. Originally, she was slated to go six or eight cycles, but since she's tolerated it so amazingly well, and had such positive results, the doctors may decide to have her go a bit longer. She told me she wouldn't mind, since that would increase the likelihood that surgery would be delayed past the middle of September. She'd prefer that, because all her various Garden Clubs have important meetings in the first two weeks of the month. When I suggested she might have her priorities a bit off, she just gave me one of those looks.

One of the other patients was having a small party at the chemo lab. It was her last session, and she had several friends and family members who came bearing balloons and a life-sized cardboard cutout of Elvis Presley. Naturally, we were all happy for her. She has maintained an impressively spunky, upbeat attitude, and wears her baseball cap jauntily. I was glad that Jeanelle wasn't there, though. She is a tall, graceful woman with fine white hair, who has carried herself with a quiet dignity. She has also steadily declined physically, so much so that the last time I saw her, I thought we wouldn't be seeing her much longer. These two women define the spectrum of cancer, its effects and treatments.

#

It is truly a life or death struggle. We're pleased that Mary seems likely to land on the life end of the spectrum, but mortality remains an ever-present specter. In fact, it reared its ugly head in a most personal manner yesterday morning, when Matthew called from Tucson, where he had been awakened at 5:30 by a phone call from the Forum, Mary's mother's assisted living center. Many of you have already heard, and the rest of you are no doubt guessing the news correctly. Matthew had the unpleasant task of informing us that Mary's mother had passed away during the night.

He sounded so awful on the phone, in so much pain, so brutally wounded, I was afraid for him. I asked if he needed to see anyone. We could call Becky, an old family friend, who was close to Mary's parents and had a great rapport with Matthew. He kept insisting he was fine, though he continued to sound awful. It was then I glanced at the clock, saw that it was 8:30. I did the math, and asked, "Do you sound so bad, because it's 5:30 in the morning?" Yes, that was the main reason, though, it was, as he texted me later, "a crappy day."

Nancy lived a good life for most of her eighty-nine years, though much of the joy went away with her husband's death nearly seven years ago. She was loving and kind, and amassed a fortune in friendships. In the last few years, attrition whittled away that lifetime's collection, so that there were not too many phone calls to be made to her contemporaries. One of her goals, her final one, was to die in her sleep, and so her life ended the way she lived it, on her terms. Now she is reunited with Val.

Mary is handling it well, having already twice said goodbye to her. She regrets not calling her Sunday night when she had the urge to, reasoning it was 7:30 in Tucson, and her mother was probably going to sleep. A missed call, never to be made now. That's something to keep in mind.

We will be flying to Tucson after chemo tomorrow, and having a small funeral service Saturday morning before returning Sunday evening. Next week starts our triumphant tour of doctors' offices, with hosannas and high fives all around, while we start to work out our strategies for the next phase.

August 19, 2010
Step Up to the Next Stage

What a frustrating day of doctors and decisions. This morning we saw Dr. Y., who told us, basically, that he wouldn't know what he was going to do until he knew what the colorectal surgeon was going to do. Dr. R., on the other hand, wasn't sure what he wanted to do, and though he was pretty confident that he would do something, he left a huge decision in Mary's lap. Which, of course, is where the decision has to be left. After all, she's the one who has to live (at least, that's the plan), with her decision.

Not only do we have to choose between an ileostomy and a colostomy, or between a low anterior recision with possible ostomy and a transanal excision, we also had to decide on the date. Would it be September 3 or September 24? There were arguments in favor of both dates, in terms of timing, travel, training, and obligations, but ultimately we decided on September 3. Guess who won't be golfing this Labor Day weekend.

Dr. Y. explained to us that the more complicated the colorectal surgery, the less likely he would be to do major liver surgery. The way things look right now, we're leaning toward the most radical surgery, as that offers the best chance for a cure. If you don't cut out the primary cancer, you'll never do more than tread water with the secondary tumors. Mary has, from the beginning, vowed to beat this thing, "to kill this thing." Which means she'll probably undergo Radiofrequency Ablation on both lobes of her liver.

It really is astounding to sit with surgeons and discuss possibilities and options, all wrapped up inside a five-to-eight-hour surgical marathon—unless the surgeons find things are worse than they expected, at which point they'll just sew her back up, and we'll move on to Plan B—so blithely tossing out possibilities and scenarios as if they didn't all have mortality as the underlying narrative.

So we're set, as of right now, for surgery on September 3. Here's the best-case scenario: Surgery followed by four to six weeks of recovery, followed by four to six weeks of chemotherapy and radiation, followed by four to six months of chemo, followed by six to eight weeks of recovery, followed, if we're lucky, by another surgery.

The good news? We might have to put that Australia trip off 'til next fall.

It's been a whirlwind month since I last sent an update, filled with visits and boat rides and plane trips and more visits with old friends and new, here, Up North, in Vermont. And it isn't over yet. Tomorrow, we're off to East Tawas for a day, to spend with one of Mary's college roommates, who married a guy from Bay City. Mary drives home Saturday, while I will be riding my bike along the Lake Huron coastline back to Grosse Pointe. I'll get back on Tuesday, just missing Mary, who will be flying to Tucson about two hours before I get home.

The social schedule has been exhausting, at least for me, the ostensibly healthy one. Mary has taken it, as she's taken just about everything else in this affair, in stride. Basically, we've packed a lifetime of travel and friends into two short months, just in case.

In some ways, the hard part is about to begin. Thanks for all your support, your love, prayers, cards, and letters. Keep it up. It means more than you can ever know.

August 31, 2010
Scheduling Conflicts

Mary's surgery has been postponed until September 24. This is mainly due to her acknowledging her Scottish roots and seeking to save time and money by having both surgeries at once. Actually, that was the plan all along, but it turns out the 24th is the first day both surgeons are free. At first Dr. A., Mary's oncologist, was not thrilled with the delay. It was too long to be optimal. Ideally, the surgery would take place on the 3rd, or sometime the following week. In the end, though, he didn't see it as a major cause for concern.

The delay actually gave us some time to do some serious rethinking of the whole affair. Paul, our oncologist friend, called with some alternative ideas, which led to the unusual experience of sitting by the side of the road somewhere near Au Gres (on our way to East Tawas), and talking on speaker phone with him. The reception kept going in and out, so we stopped in a live zone.

Paul's idea, which represents some of the cutting-edge thinking coming out of Houston's MD Anderson, is to focus on the liver first. This is the complete opposite of everything we've been hearing, which is to get rid of the primary cancer before it can spread further. This alternative targets the liver, because that's the cancer that can kill, while holding the rectal tumor at bay with radiation. In a nutshell, if you can't control the liver, why put the patient through the inconvenience and possible ignominy of a colostomy?

It gave us something to think about, and some time in which to do it. The main thing we realized, is that this new approach, with its Plan B quality, and its palliative nature, implies a sense of giving in to cancer. In Mary's eyes, and in mine, giving in sounds a lot like giving up. It's the same with her preferring the inconvenience and potential complications of an ileostomy over the relative simplicity of a colostomy. Anything less than going after a cure is surrender.

We have friends who have faced multiple bouts with cancer, and are still here to talk about it, and to encourage us. It is a great resource for Mary to talk with people who are authorities by virtue of their still walking the planet.

Sadly, we also saw cancer claim new victims. A friend lost her son, too soon, too much younger than we are. Then shortly after, Peter, husband to one of Mary's oldest friends from Tucson, fell, after a long, furious, heroic battle which he should have and could have lost years ago. Now Mary's trying to work out a time to go visit her. And that's one good outcome of the delay.

Another was that Mary got to go out to Tucson last week, to finish dealing with her mother's affairs. While she was gone, I rode my bike down from East Tawas to Grosse Pointe. I spent a lot of time on the bike questioning my motives, wondering if this trip was simply a matter of running away. Was it in some sense a betrayal? I had to answer in the negative. It's what I've done every year for a decade now, and I already shifted the timing several times to accommodate Mary's scheduling needs. Plus I needed it for my mental health. And finally, Mary didn't mind.

So I rode, and survived, and started cleaning out the basement while Mary was gone. Now we're looking at three weeks, which no doubt will fly past. We'll continue working out, and getting in shape. I'll keep you posted, and though things still could change, right now we're set for the 24th.

September 14, 2010
We'll Get By With a Little Help From Our Friends

With ten days to go until surgery, it's time for some housekeeping. Our friend, Mary Beth, has set up a page called "Lend Mary a Hand," at a website called "Lotsa Helping Hands." One of the main features of this site is a calendar, on which we can list things we might need, be it a meal, a ride, or just company. Not knowing how Mary will respond to surgery, we don't know how extensive her needs will be, but the site provides a resource both for us and for our friends who want to help. It eliminates the problem of too much help when it isn't needed, and not enough when it is.

As I understand it, you need to join the community if you want to offer yourself as a resource. Granted, this doesn't really apply to those of you who aren't local, but I thought it was easier to just include this information in an update.

One the community is populated, we will be able to post a need to the calendar, and you will be notified. Once someone responds, that need is no longer outstanding. This is all new to me, so we will have to see how it goes, but Mary Beth said one of her sisters used it when she had cancer, and it was literally a lifesaver.

I was just humming the words to that old Beatles song, to which the title of this piece alludes, and I started to laugh. "When I'm Sixty-Four?" It doesn't seem that long ago that sixty-four seemed a lifetime away. Not so much anymore. Of course getting there is what this is all about now.

We're ten days away from surgery. I don't know how Mary's doing, but I'm a wreck. I mentioned to a friend I was having trouble sleeping, being frequently awakened by vivid dreams detailing various obstacles to my getting Mary to the hospital for surgery. He noted that was no doubt a reflection of my feeling helpless. There is some truth to that. I can help support her, do what I can to encourage her, and after surgery, do whatever it takes to help her recover, but at the end of the day this is a matter for Mary first of all, and then the abilities of her surgeons. If something goes wrong with either of those factors, I can have the best attitude in the world, and the most selfless intentions, and they will mean nothing.

So we move forward. The reason I don't know how Mary is doing is she has spent the last few days in Oklahoma, with her friend Cordelia, the loss of whose husband I mentioned in the last update. Peter fought cancer for twenty years, which is pretty amazing. Cordelia told me, "We had twenty years to plan Peter's funeral, and we never said one word about it." Mary just called, waiting for her return flight, and said the visit was good. It was important for her to be there. Important for Cordelia, and also for herself, I'm sure. The best way to avoid hearing the footsteps is to keep moving.

Back in 2005, after dropping Matthew at the University of Arizona, we went on what we called our Empty Nest Road Trip. We drove back to Michigan from Tucson by way of California, where we visited my family and our friends throughout the state, including Cordelia and Peter, who at that time lived in Ben Lomond, in the redwood drenched hills above Santa Cruz. Peter's cancer, which pretty much had free rein in his body, had recently moved to his tongue, which necessitated the removal of about half of it.

As we approached their home, my instinctive coward's reflex arose, and all I wanted to do was run away. But no, I resolved, not this time. This time I would be a man, and I was, and I asked Peter about his cancer, about the adjustment to losing so much of his tongue. And he spoke, painfully, slowly, but at length about the challenges he was facing. At that time I had no idea that one day we would be facing similar challenges, but it was a first step to responsibility.

After surgery, Mary will be in the hospital for four to seven days. When she comes home, we will be in an unfamiliar country. Neither of us has any experience with invasive surgery, so we really don't know what the recovery process will entail. One thing we do know, though, is for the first time since our adventure began, Mary will definitely be sick. That's where my work will begin. It's easy to be a supportive cancer spouse when the full extent of your duties are to coordinate her visitors and her travels. Now, though, things will be different.

This is where our friends come in, because, folks keep telling me, this is where I'll need help. Curiously, my initial reaction to talk of coordinating schedules for food, and care, and company, was one of resistance. I'm not one of those husbands who is helpless in the kitchen, the type of guy who might starve if his wife isn't there to cook for him. I wasn't sure how much help we were going to need, and I definitely didn't like the idea of being shunted off to the side. But gradually others have convinced me of the importance of taking a day or two a week off, and to rely on others to prepare dinner and offer company, as needed.

(You may find it interesting that Mary has been one of the strongest advocates of my taking time out for myself. Rather than an indication of concern for my well being, I suspect this has more to do with her dread of being restricted to her bed, unable to escape my jokes, my humorous, fact-based anecdotes, my creative reminiscences, or my cogent, insightful analyses of world affairs and domestic politics).

So as we approach the border of this forbidding new territory, the customs agents all wear white coats, with white gloves on their hands–unless you have an allergy to latex. They don't ask you why you've come and how long you intend to stay, but they make it plain, in the kindest possible manner, that they hope you go back home, soon.

September 23, 2010
Pulling Weeds

Our yard was infested with Gill Over the Ground, a highly invasive ground cover which spreads via runners. Also known as Creeping Charlie, if left untended, it can completely overwhelm a lawn. While small concentrations can be controlled through hand weeding, we were advised that herbicides were our best option.

A couple weeks ago, I took it upon myself to eradicate the pest by hand. Mary suggested it was therapeutic, and I think she was right. The other day, I was sprawled on the lawn, pulling strands of grass apart as I uprooted runners as long as two feet in length. In the process, I pulled up some grass, and left huge bare patches in the lawn, where the weeds had completely taken over. By the time I finished, the lawn looked far worse than when I had started, which meant I had to put down new topsoil and grass seed, and hope it takes root before winter comes.

This, I realized, is a lot like fighting cancer. Our surgeons and oncologists are trying to uproot this highly invasive species, and in the process, they're uprooting good tissue as well. Cancer treatment has come a long, long way, but in its essence, it is still a race to destroy the cancer before you destroy the body. Once removed, we can plant new seeds and work to recreate the healthy landscape which existed before the invasion.

I know I was successful in stopping Creeping Charlie's advance. I also know I will have to remain vigilant next spring and in the coming years to inspect the lawn, and to act at the first sign of its return. In the same way, with Mary, if the uprooting is successful, she will undergo frequent tests in the future to make sure it doesn't return.

Things have proceeded swimmingly for the past six months. Mary's health has been surprisingly good. She has tolerated her treatments, and we just finished what was, in so many ways, one of the best summers of our lives. But now the serious uprooting begins. Henry Ford Hospital just called, to inform us we need to arrive at 5:30 tomorrow morning. Surgery is scheduled to begin at 7:00. If all goes well, it will go on for several hours.

We are no longer playing at make-believe. In less than twenty-four hours the landscape of our lives will be completely disrupted, and the task of healing will begin in earnest. The last two weeks of not knowing have been hard, harder it seems, on me than on Mary. Maybe because she has a deeper well of inner strength, or a more placid outlook on life and its possibilities.

The way she spent her day is a compelling example of the equanimity with which she faces her challenge. She had a hair appointment today, because, of course, everyone wants to look good for their surgeons. Then she decided it would be fun to invite some friends to come along for manicures, pedicures, and facials.

What better way to get ready for surgery than a Spa Party?

Emily flew in on the Red Eye from Sacramento yesterday, and will drive back west one day next week to begin her classes a couple weeks late. Matthew, though willing to come, is racing against time in a bid to complete his undergrad studies by January. We told him to stay in Arizona. Thanksgiving break will be here soon enough. Better to reflect Dr. Y.'s philosophy, that this is no big deal. A few hours under the knife, and then we're back on our way. After all, it's not like it's rocket surgery or anything, just a simple procedure involving a rectum, a liver, and two surgeons.

We appreciate everyone's prayers and support, and want to thank the dozens of friends who have signed up to "Lend Mary a Hand." We'll let you know what Mary needs, and when she needs it. I'll post something tomorrow night to let you know how the surgery went, and what the prospects are for visiting.

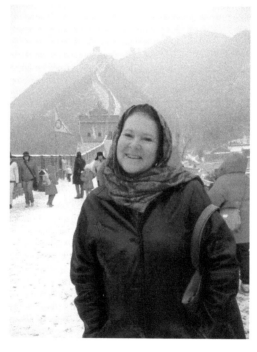

Mary on the Great Wall of China. In 2006 she took Emily on a trip around the world to celebrate her graduation from Cornell, University.
—Photo by Emily Goodell

September 24, 2010
She Can Hit the Curveball

A couple of updates back I mentioned how our friend Paul threw a curveball into our plans, suggesting an alternative approach to surgery. His idea was to focus first on the liver cancer, since that was the cancer that could kill. After a flurry of discussions, and second-guessing, and rethinking, we, and our surgeons, with Paul's concurrence, decided to stick with our original plan.

Imagine our surprise then, when Emily and I were summoned to the waiting room desk after about an hour. We were directed into the hallway where Dr. R. stood. Before we could say a word, he said, "It's not what you think," which showed good sense on his part, because everyone has heard the story of so-and-so who went in for surgery, but when they opened him up they saw there was nothing they could do, so they just sewed him right back up again. And that's what you think has happened when the surgeon is standing around in the hallway one hour into a six-hour procedure.

That wasn't the case here, the surgeon assured us. Instead, during the laparoscopic probe, they discovered a couple of things. One, the cancer had not spread through the pelvic region, which was good news. Two, there was no sign of cancer in the left lobe of the liver. The right one, though, had three tumors. After detailed discussion, the surgeons agreed that, instead of doing the Low Anterior Resection and removing the left lobe of the liver with RFA on the tumors on the right, Dr. Y. would remove the right lobe. This is a much more complex surgery than removing the left, and because of the stress on the body, it mitigated against doing the rectal surgery.

In other words, once they saw what they were dealing with, they decided to go with the curveball. After Mary recovers from this surgery, she will undergo two or three more months of chemo, along with radiation. Then, maybe four months from now, she will undergo further surgery, to remove the rectal tumor. This has a couple of advantages. One, she won't have to deal with an ileostomy or colostomy while recovering from this major surgery. Two, one of the risks involved in doing chemo after the resection was the inhibiting effect it would have on healing the tissues. This increases the chances of success for that surgery. (Plus, as an added bonus, Dr. R. determined it was possible to attach the colon to the sphincter, which means Mary could have a temporary ileostomy, and not be saddled with a permanent colostomy).

But that is further down the road. First comes recovery. This was major, major surgery, and it took more than six hours to complete. By the time Mary left the recovery room and was installed in her own room, we had been at the hospital for more than thirteen hours. By the time we got in to see her, all she wanted to do was sleep. Which is how we left her. We'll go back tomorrow, planning to spend the day.

At this point, I'm not sure whether non-family visitors are even allowed, though certainly, she isn't up to receiving them anyway. I'll let you know if this changes after the weekend. We don't know when she will be coming home, as it is, of course, very early in the recovery process. The important thing to know is Mary survived the surgery. She came out of it in very good shape. She was coherent, and miserable, and ready to move on to the next stage.

#

Last Thursday night we had visitors, Bruce and Nancy from Toronto, and Denis and Janey from Boston. That was a total of three cancer survivors, which was not a bad sendoff for surgery. The ride to the hospital, at 5:00 this morning, was as tense as you might imagine. But we were armed with the support of friends, and the preop process was filled with laughter and love.

Emily was there, with her friend, Laura. Kate came in later, with a dozen bagels, and Cindy dropped by in the afternoon. From our contemporaries, Margaret, Izzy, and Laura, aka "Nine," were there. They kept things light, and fun, and we all supported each other during the seemingly interminable wait. Best news of all? The waiting room was divided between a room with televisions and a designated quiet area. The quiet area was anything but, filled with laughter, conversation, and groups huddled together to share their affections.

Our world did change today, in a manner different than we expected. We have a new game plan, one which I am confident Mary will execute as successfully as the last ones. We're moving ahead with renewed hope, and the comfort and confidence inspired by the love and support of friends too numerous to count.

September 28, 2010
Walking Cancer Down the Hall

Mary and I were strolling down the hallway outside her room Sunday afternoon, she with her hand resting on my crooked arm, for security rather than support. We moved at a gentle, almost serene pace, like some mutant Seurat painting of perambulating Parisians, the other patrons dressed in matching blue or white scrubs, and the duck pond replaced with darkened rooms inhabited by people slowly coming back to life, or trying to retain their hold on it. If that scene weren't bizarre enough, I was reminded of some of the lyrics from Tom Waits' song, "Walking Spanish Down the Hall."

Walking Spanish is slang for the act of escorting someone by the nape of his neck and the seat of his pants, synonymous with giving one the bum's rush. Which I guess is what this massive, invasive surgery was all about, an unceremonious eviction of the interloping cancer. In the days to come, we shall see how effective that strategy has been.

When Dr. Y. came in to see Mary Saturday, the day after surgery, he cried "You look fantastic!" A glance at the surprise in his eyes upon seeing her proved that his enthusiasm wasn't just for show. She looked surprisingly well, and her physical condition was also beyond expectation. We all thought it was good news when he said she would probably go home Tuesday, "if not Monday."

The nurses' goal for her that first day was to get her out of bed twice, and to sit in a chair for an hour or two. Her first walk down the hall was her idea, and the staff was highly supportive in their approval. Sunday, Mary was up almost as often as she was down. Her spirits were good, and she ate a larger portion of her meals, and things were definitely looking up when I left.

Then came yesterday. Not a good day as these things go. Physically, Mary is continuing to improve. In fact, by the time Emily and I got there almost all the various iv's, catheters, and other mysterious tubes had been removed from her body. She had already been up and walking unassisted three times, and the night before had repeatedly gotten out of bed without any help. Yet Mary felt miserable, and there was nothing anyone could do to make her feel better.

It wasn't really pain, more a general discomfort, and a horrible bloated, gassy feeling. I told her it that was natural, since her insides had undergone such terrible trauma just two days before. She was, however, basically inconsolable, and began talking about having to stay in the hospital until Friday, if not through the following weekend.

I think mainly what she was feeling was depression, which, given the seriousness of the surgery, and the range of drugs coursing through her blood—not to mention they took away her morphine button—seems like a natural outcome. Of course Mary, not being subject to depression, has a little trouble recognizing it. If it were me, I'd know who depression was while he was walking up the sidewalk. I'd meet him at the door, usher him in. "Grab a chair, sit down, take a load off." Mary doesn't have that luxury, and was not at all pleased when they told her last night she'll probably be going home today.

I'm heading down to the hospital now, and hope she's

feeling better. I wonder if hospitals should focus exclusively on physical recuperation in this sort of situation? Surely the emotional component is almost as important in achieving a satisfactory recovery. Even if Mary were physically able to do cartwheels down the hall, would she be ready for release if she thought her body was about to explode? Well, we shall see what her condition is today, and whether anyone has changed their mind.

I'll send out a blurb this afternoon to let you know if she is at home. At that point, we'll fire up the Lend Mary a Hand website, and stuff the calendar with increasingly more shrill and unreasonable demands.

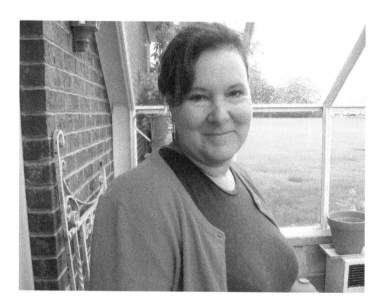

September 28, 2010
Sometimes It Rains

Today was a lousy day to drive to the hospital. A steady rain was falling, the kind that lays on the freeways allowing every truck to create its own impermeable weather system. While driving, alternately accelerating out of trouble then braking to avoid the next spin out, and trying to figure out what it is about inclement weather that makes people think, "This looks like a good day to forget everything I ever knew about operating a motor vehicle," I wondered what the day would bring. How would Mary feel today? Would her spirits be better? Is she more comfortable with the idea of going home? Has that gaseous, bloated feeling begun to ease?

When I got there, she was hooked back up to an IV, and a nurse was telling her the tests were scheduled for 1:00. It turns out she had a bad night, very little sleep, bad nausea. She's back on a liquid diet while they determine whether there are intestinal problems. In short, she won't be coming home today. She is still getting stronger, though, and her hallway walks are getting faster and faster. So this is just a setback, an understandable complication, but nothing that should inhibit a proper recovery.

When Emily showed up around 1:30, as they were wheeling Mary to the X-Ray department, I headed out into the deluge to buy a reclining lift chair. What an exciting lifestyle breakthrough! Unfortunately, they informed me that I couldn't get it in Naugahyde, as naugas are now listed as an endangered species. I decided to forego the beverage holder option. No doubt when Mary is fully recovered, and I rescind my NFL boycott, that decision will come back to haunt me.

I'll keep you informed. You can always call me on my cell during visiting hours, and I'll check to see if Mary feels up to talking with you.

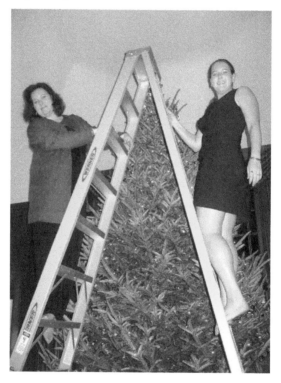

Celebrating Christmas was a huge part of Mary's year. Here she poses with Emily in front of the annual 15-foot tree.

September 30, 2010
Moving Day

It looks like Mary will be coming home today. The tests they ran the other day were negative, her nausea is gone, she's back on solid foods, and her system is tolerating it. Plus, she got the lab results which showed only one of the three tumors in the right lobe was cancerous, and the one small lesion in the left lobe, which remains in her body, was not cancerous. So, right now, her liver is cancer-free.

In a few weeks, we'll resume chemo and begin radiation treatments, and after that, once more under the knife. As our friend Paul put it the other day, "Mary is one operation away from being in remission." Considering where we started, that is an incredible result.

Of course, we don't want to be guilty of engaging in a premature poultry population assessment, but there is every reason for optimism at this point. Now, off to Helping Hands to lay out a series of demands, then down to Henry Ford Hospital, for the last time in quite awhile.

Perhaps, it's not a moment too soon. Yesterday, when I went to visit, I got on the elevator and pressed 6 as usual.

However, when I reached the sixth floor, nothing happened. For a moment, that is, because instead of the door opening, the elevator started to fall. It stopped at the third floor, though the doors remained shut. Fortunately, when I pressed the open button, they complied. I hopped off, waited, pressed the call button and boarded a different elevator to the top. But it seems a reasonable rule that when the elevators turn against you, it's time to go home.

October 5, 2010
Circle the Wagons

Lately, I've started feeling like Gary Cooper or Randolph Scott in one of those old Hollywood westerns. The ones where they circle the wagon train and everyone holds their positions, rifle at the ready, waiting for the indigenous peoples to register their displeasure with the illegal immigrants in their midst. Cooper says to Scott, "It's quiet out there," and Scott replies, "Yeah——too quiet."

Mary handled her surgery about as well as she's handled everything else in the last six months. Aside from that one blip last Tuesday, her recovery was ahead of schedule. Dr. Y. dropped in last Thursday, just before Mary was discharged, to tell her she was about the best patient he'd ever seen. Our ride home was punctuated with heavy traffic, and a large number of drivers exhibiting substandard motoring skills. At one point, as we avoided another mishap, Mary murmured, "Wouldn't that be ironic."

As I had some post-discharge errands to run, we arranged for Laura to meet us at the house. When I returned, I found Mary making her friend some tea. She stood in the kitchen as she went through the twenty or so cards and care packages that had accumulated. Meanwhile, I savored my one piece of mail, a "Thank You" card from Janis, the salesclerk at the furniture store where I bought the recliner.

The next morning, Mary got up and made her own breakfast. The next evening, we went for a half-mile walk. Yesterday she stretched it out to a mile, made her own lunch, and dropped in at the Herb Society Board Meeting in the afternoon. It isn't a case of pushing things, though. She gets tired in the evening, and sleeps in most mornings, and is happy to have things done for her. But the sense I had before surgery, that now the fun times were over, and we were going to learn what it was like to be really sick, that hasn't happened.

It's uncanny. So much so that I've started to wonder, can it really be this easy? Can we have gone from a statistical death sentence, and a doctor saying there was no prospect of surgery, "We'll do chemo and hope it works," to a situation where we are looking total remission in the eyes and are not even tempted to blink? All in the space of just six short months? It's quiet. Too quiet.

Of course, there's still another course of chemo, this time with radiation, and then another major surgery in three or four months, so it's not like Mary's ready to start training for a marathon or anything like that. (Though Sunday morning she suggested we might ride our bikes up to Provencal. I demurred, pointing to the risks of her falling off). Still, Mary has handled everything they've thrown at her, and this includes the diagnosis, with aplomb. It's been inspirational to be around her, not just for me, but for so many of our friends as well.

I'll keep you posted on Mary's progress. Please continue to call and write, and shower her with love, and help us continue, each day, to be dazzled by the transcendent power of friendship and prayer

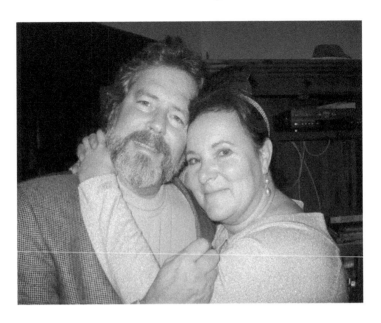

October 20, 2010
Born to It

Back when Mary was thriving while pregnant with our first child, I remarked in jest that she was born to be pregnant. She was not amused, my quip smacking of kitchens and unshod feet. The other day I made a similar comment, that she seemed to have been born to have cancer. I didn't mean it as a joke. It just blurted out when we were talking with friends about how amazing her experience has been.

After the paralyzing fear and dismay which followed the diagnosis and confirmation of Stage 4 cancer, once we began the process, it was surprisingly easy, with few side effects and strongly positive results. Of course, we knew, once she had her surgery, things would change. And yet they haven't. The hard times haven't come. Just about an hour ago our friend Laura referred to Mary's recovery as "miraculous."

That's not an inaccurate description. Sometimes it is hard to believe it was just a little over three weeks ago that she had sixty percent of her liver removed, along with her gallbladder. I've been telling people she's about eighty percent, which means she could play quarterback right now, but we'd like to hold her out until after the bye week. She is off on an errand right now, delivering a car full of dried plants to the location of this year's Herb Society crafts workshop. Tomorrow we're driving down to Ohio for a funeral, and the day after we're off to Saugatuck to visit Chuck and Ruth, then up to Glen Lake for a few days. The trip Up North, though probably too late to see many fall colors, is still an exciting prospect, as we had assumed there wouldn't be a fall trip on our itinerary this year.

Mary has been walking up to four miles a day. She has a green light to drive. She is cooking most dinners herself (apparently, I had overestimated my culinary skills). Sometimes it almost seems like this whole thing has been a fiction, as if we were perpetrating a fraud on friends and family. (Incidentally, there should be a special level of hell for the people who do do that). On the other hand, Mary has a ten-inch scar on her belly which helps deflect any suspicions along those lines.

Last Friday, we met Lincoln and Mary Beth at the Detroit Art Institute to hear a jazz piano concert by George Winston. (I suggested maybe we could stop by the Music Hall afterwards, to look at some paintings). The concert, which took place in the Rivera Court, was heavily attended, as free concerts tend to be, with every chair taken, every inch of space occupied by standees, and an overflow area in the Great Hall next door serviced by a video feed.

At one point in the concert, one of the standing women collapsed. She was off to the side and toward the back, and she fell silently, so only those nearest to her, and a few observant others, even knew what had happened. The pianist was unaware, and continued to play while a doctor knelt over the prostrate form and rendered aid. The thing ended happily as she quickly recovered and walked away under her own power. Still, while the scene unfolded, I reflected on how aptly it reflected our lives. How insignificant our individual issues become within the broad spectrum of existence. Life marches on, unyieldingly, ignorant of our starring performance in our own compelling drama.

Which is as it should be, and we should be ever cognizant of how inconsequential our place is on the planet. Yet, within that small circle, there is nothing inconsequential. The lessons we have learned, the love and kindnesses which have been showered upon us, and the prayers sent heavenward by Christians, Jews, Hindus and even atheists have been overwhelming. It's so great to feel a part of a winning team.

We're rounding the final turn, and heading down the finishing stretch now. There is still some heavy lifting to do though, and more challenges lie ahead. The last week of October will be filled with doctors' visits and further diagnostic tests. The following week it looks like Mary will begin a five-week course of chemo and radiation therapy. She's rather pleased with the timing, as it will end in time for the Christmas holidays and festivities.

Some time after the new year, Mary will undergo another major surgery, to remove her rectum, and some months after that, a final, more routine operation will reattach everything inside. From that point forward, we will have the opportunity to live cancer-free. Whether it turns out that way, is of course, anybody's guess. At best, we will have donated a full year out of our lives to enact our own personal drama, off to the side while the pianist continued to pound the keys.

Going forward, Mary will face regular tests and exams, each of which will no doubt be fraught with uncertainty. What if it comes back? What if it is worse this time? What if it finally starts to hurt? Only time will tell, but I'm pretty confident that between those tests and bouts of doubt, we will be living life to the best of our abilities. As the saying goes, "Living well is the best revenge."

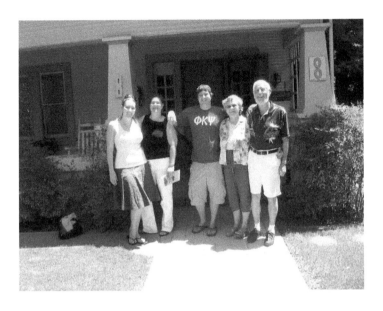

Family was of preeminent value to Mary. Here she poses with her children and Michael's parents, Martha and Malcolm Goodell, in Lodi, California

November 9, 2010
Confessions of a Supernumerary

Lately I've been caught by surprise when people ask about Mary. Wherever I go friends approach, and with that profoundly sincere expression, ask, "How is Mary doing?" I respond, reflexively, "Fine," while wondering why the special emphasis. Then I catch up with reality and realize, of course, it's because she has cancer.

I confess I don't spend a lot of time these days thinking about Mary's cancer. When we make plans for tomorrow, next month, and next year, we no longer do it with the proviso, "If." If she's up to it. If she's able to travel. If she's still around, we'll do this or go there. We just make plans based on the assumption that she will be.

It's a remarkable change in our outlook. Or perhaps I should say my outlook. It's entirely possible that Mary is more conversant with her status as a cancer patient. After all, she's the one going to chemo each Monday to have her five-day pump installed, and each Friday to have it removed. She's the one going to radiation Monday through Friday. She's the one getting blood tests and platelet counts and CEA scores. She's also the one who will undergo another major surgery, probably in January.

#

The fact is, though, that this bout of chemo and radiation doesn't seem to be slowing her down at all. They warned her that it would probably make her tired. Never averse to napping, she didn't see that as necessarily being a negative. However, if anything, she seems to have more energy. On the other hand, we were also warned that the effects of radiation are cumulative, and we're only in the second of five weeks, so perhaps we shouldn't be giving high fives just yet.

Beginning last Wednesday, I haven't even taken Mary to radiation. That was the day she told me I didn't need to take her, because she was going to a Garden Club Luncheon immediately after her session. (That was also the day after I was caught berating the receptionists, saying "You mean if I don't want to watch 'The View' I have to go sit in the chapel?"). The next day, it was shopping, right after radiation.

I'm not needed. That's a strange position in which to find myself. Then again, it's been a strange situation for the past eight months. I was thinking the other day how naturally immersed we have become in the world of cancer. It happened all at once, one otherwise normal day back in early March. Then the world changed, irrevocably and immediately. What struck me though, was how quickly we adapted to our new world. How quickly cancer became the new normal.

Now, obviously, Mary still has cancer, and she still has a lot of work ahead of her. What I find interesting is the way we're starting to let down our guard. Sometimes I caution myself not to be so cavalier, not to start to assume the best, not to fall under the sway of hubris. But from right here, in this place, on this day, things are looking good. We look back on those long odds we faced, and we're starting to think, "Yeah, that was a good bet."

Let's keep in touch. Mary's fighting like a hero, but she

still needs and appreciates your support. (And I do, too, especially those of you who have made the effort to include me in your expressions of concern, and of support).

December 7, 2010
Thankful for Thanksgiving

With the exception of the week immediately following her surgery, the past two weeks have probably been the hardest Mary has faced. This might come as a surprise to those of you who have spent any time with her during that period. The fact that she did everything on her calendar, including cooking Thanksgiving Dinner for seven (with a big assist from Emily and her friends, Shreya and Swetcha), and hosting forty or so for that Saturday's Tree Trimming Party, reinforces what I've come to understand. Mary is a very strong person.

It's one thing to seemingly waltz through the entire experience, to look Stage 4 in the eye and wait for cancer to blink, to never have symptoms and never get sick. It's quite another when you do feel sick. When it hurts to stand and it hurts to sit, and your bathroom looks like a MASH unit for all the hemorrhoid pads, lotions, and unguents scattered around, that is when you decide whether you want to step up to the plate.

It's one of the side effects of radiation, they say, so Mary has been trying to accept the fact that she isn't entirely immune to the whole experience. I reminded her the other day that we were expecting, and had expected for more than eight months for her to suffer. So in a way, suffering helps us both appreciate again what a wonderful gift we've been given in the months which went before.

And as I said, Mary's suffering hasn't really slowed her down. Granted, yesterday she didn't feel up to going out to Somerset with me to do some Christmas shopping. It was a tough blow for me, but being a trouper, I bravely accepted the fact that we wouldn't spend the evening in a shopping mall.

Mary is in her final week of chemo and radiation, and then we'll wait six or eight weeks before surgery. No doubt there will be another CT scan, though we don't know for sure. The ball will soon be in Dr. R.'s court, and we'll go where he tells us. If all goes well with surgery, by the beginning of March, Mary will be cancer free, and we will look back on a full year taken from us, but also at the gifts life has given us during that year. Then the challenge will be to remember the lessons learned, and to keep at the forefront of our minds the value inherent in life and the obligation to live it to the fullest.

This is shaping up to be a completely different holiday season for me. For years my mood has turned south at the first sight of goblins, ghouls, and jack-o-lanterns, as Halloween heralded the start of another long, overindulgent and obligation-filled season. Somehow, this year, I haven't had my usual brush with despair. You might argue that it's early, there's still plenty of time for my seasonal depression to set in. Somehow, I don't think it will happen this year. When we sat down to the groaning board this past Thanksgiving, and I offered, as annually obligated, a Thanksgiving prayer, I began by thanking God for the gift of life, and I meant it, and mean it. It's a great gift. We need to always remember that.

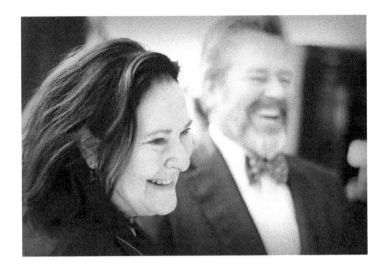

Photographer Unknown.

December 31, 2010
We'll Get There

Put a tick mark next to the latest milestone. We finished the year. I wouldn't have given you good odds on that one back in March, when our world came crashing down. But there you have it. The miracle of life, the power of prayer, and the wonders of modern medicine combined to create the greatest Christmas gift possible.

Having both kids home made it special. Opening their gifts to us made me stop and think how thoughtful their presents were, and to wonder how on earth we managed to convey that message to them. We exchanged gifts, we went to late church, where Mary sang in the choir, and we passed the flame and sang "Silent Night" by candlelight, and what a Holy moment that was.

The week before we had flown to Arizona where we met up with Emily and my parents, and watched Matthew graduate from the University. He was proud, and so were we, and relieved, and excited about the new career he is careening toward in New Orleans. Funny how sometimes people grow up suddenly. At times I wonder how much Mary's illness contributed to his turning the corner so abruptly.

Mary was still feeling the effects of radiation when we flew to Tucson. She was uncomfortable, and often in pain, and I responded at times with impatience. It reminded me of what my job is here, to give her the care and support she so badly needs. Only, of course, as you may have gathered from these reports, demand for those duties was in short supply over the previous nine months. Mary handled the procedures and treatments so well that I grew complacent. Only in the past month has she been sick, and it has been a revelation. As she struggles now, I am all the more amazed at how well she has done.

When we returned, we had our annual Christmas party, with some fifty or so people passing through the house and staying as late as they wished. It was a wonderful time, and everyone kept remarking how well Mary looked. And she did. She's lost a bit of weight from the last bout of chemo and radiation, and it reflects nicely on her. You may recall after the first chemo session she complained that she hadn't lost weight.

Lately, Mary is having good days and bad days. Christmas Eve was a good day. Christmas Day was not. She asked if we minded if she didn't cook Christmas Dinner. No, we didn't mind. We could have tried it ourselves, but she wanted to do it, and she didn't feel like eating it that day if we did manage to make it. The next day, she was fine, and we had our Christmas Dinner one day late.

The question we confront now is what is causing this discomfort. It's hard to know, without further testing, because the region where the radiation was focused, is, naturally the region where the cancer remains. Is Mary's discomfort simply a side effect, or is it a sign that the radiation didn't work? That's a hard question to ask, and, though we hope for the best, I fear the worst sort of answer.

Sometimes it feels as if we've been abandoned by the medical profession. We've passed from one side, treatment, to the next, surgery. Only the surgeon isn't ready to see us.

That will happen on the 13th. Then what? Is a physical exam enough, or do we need another CT Scan? If the latter, will there be enough time to schedule it before the optimal time for surgery passes? What about blood tests? Shouldn't someone be checking for CEA or any other markers? Is there something I was supposed to do which I forgot about?

The questions are the hardest part, and the fear that things are no longer going as well as they have been, and as we have said they have been going.

This morning I read an email from our friends Nigel and Sabine, wondering if we were planning to visit England any time soon, or if they should plan to come over here next year. I wrote back to say we didn't know what our plans were. We weren't sure when we would be going to Australia, though probably it would be next fall, and if we would come back via Europe if we did. I said "It's hard to make plans when you don't know what the future holds, or it's easy to make plans when you don't know what the future holds. On the one hand, you can't really commit, on the other, you can commit to everything knowing you possibly won't or can't do anything."

And that's pretty much where we stand at this point, on the precipice of a New Year, ready and willing to face the challenges that lie ahead, eager to embrace the victories, unsettled at times by the uncertainties, but grateful for the love and support and prayers of friends near and far.

Happy New Year.

January 11, 2011
Down the Home Stretch

It feels like the end of something, this final ten days before what we hope will be the penultimate surgery in Mary's saga. Yes, it is scheduled for the 21st. If all goes well, it should take several hours. Mary's spirits are good, and she is feeling better than she was when I sent my last update. Of course, this is very encouraging. You may recall the concern before was whether her pain and discomfort were side effects of radiation therapy, or were they a sign that the treatment wasn't working, that the cancer was continuing to grow. It was hard to tell since the symptoms would have been the same.

However, she has continued to feel better over the past two weeks. She's not one hundred percent, but she is feeling better for longer periods of time. In fact, her not feeling good now is the anomaly. This is encouraging, because I've got to believe if her discomfort was caused by the cancer, she would continue to feel worse, and not better. No doubt Dr. R. will help shed some light on this subject Thursday afternoon.

If all goes well, we hope to head up to Glen Lake on Friday. Not really a last hurrah, but it will be the last time we'll have that freedom for a while. Our post-surgery goal is to head back Up North for President's Day Weekend. Emily has booked her flights for that time. She won't be here for surgery, as classes intrude. Matthew won't be either as he'll be in the process of moving to New Orleans for post-graduate employment. It's okay this time. We will have friends around to distract me from my default morbidity, and our sense of drama and foreboding at this surgical go-round are greatly reduced.

Which is why we've set the ambitious travel goal. In part, it reflects our confidence (tempered with the recognition that it remains something far more challenging than a formality, thereby forestalling dread hubris). In part, too, our goal reflects the fun we've had before at the Glen Arbor Chili Cook-Off. The competition features dozens of traditional and non-traditional chili recipes, submitted by local restaurants, taverns, stores, and individuals for judgment by hundreds of hungry, opinionated judges.

It's all in good fun, and the money raised goes to a good cause. One of the best things about the day is the pleasure of seeing hundreds of people milling about in twenty-degree temperatures, as happily as on a summer day. Everyone there is there because he or she enjoys winter. There is a kinship I find quite compelling.

That same kinship has carried us through this journey, and I am confident it will carry us the rest of the way. We were speaking with a friend after church last Sunday about the lessons we've learned along the way. Mary said in some ways getting cancer is the best thing that ever happened to her, because it has taught her what really matters. Family, friends, a sunrise, a sunset. Cancer strips away the extraneous. It helps you see more clearly than you've ever seen before, the value of a friend, the worthiness of a project or task. Traditions are either jettisoned or embraced, and in their treatment is our understanding made manifest.

#

So we move ahead with confidence, and with the hopes that

ten days from now Mary will be completely cancer-free. Of course, even if she is, she still is in line for another three months of chemotherapy. Cancer isn't sport, where there are rules against kicking someone when they're down. Cancer doesn't play by the rules, and neither will we. If we have cancer on the run, we'll run it down, and kill it.

When that is done, we've made so many plans; it's hard to decide which ones to act on first. There will be so many friends, old friendships renewed, and new friendships made incredibly vital, to be affirmed and treasured, and nurtured with visits. There are places we need to go, places we've never been and places we realize we need to return to. We have spent time, in the evening, often in bed when neither of us could sleep, just talking over memories, of places, people, vistas, and meals. Sometimes looking back can help you see the way forward.

I can't wait until this is done, when after fifteen months or so the healthcare establishment tells us we can have our lives back. In the meantime, there remains a bit of heavy lifting to do. Which means you need to pray, call, write, and all the other things you've done, which mean so much and have helped Mary, thus far, stay in the winning column. I'll be firing up the old "Mary Needs A Helping Hand" website again in the next few days, begging for meals and company. Just so you're forewarned.

January 21, 2011
What's Time to a Pig?

I've been working on this one for awhile in my head, but I realized today, driving home from the hospital, that the format I had in mind required, in journalist's parlance, burying the lede. So we'll dispense with the elegant essay and get right to "The Top Story Tonight," as "Saturday Night Live" used to put it.

We got up at 5:00 am this morning and got to the hospital by six. Into Pre-Op by 7:00, and after the usual administrative runaround, we were making progress by 8:00. Laura, Margaret, and Izzy arrived at around 7:30, and took turns, two-by-two, in the cramped pre-surgical quarters. When it was time for them to leave, they said things like, "See you on the other side," to which Mary said, "Don't say 'the other side.' to someone going into surgery." Margaret said, "Oh, I just meant on the other side of the curtain, there," gesturing at the flimsy curtain which separated our grim battle from the humdrum world of paper processing and schedule filling. Mary said, "Don't say curtains!" Which gives you an indication of her mood going in.

Upbeat, and justifiably so. Some three hours later, Dr. R. came out to give me the news. It went as well as could be hoped. He removed the tumor, and much of the rectum, but there was enough margin left, "only just," he clarified, to attach the colon. The connection was good; there were no leaks, he assured me. Mary will have an ileostomy bag for six months or so, but then we should be able to reconnect her system, and she will move ahead unhindered.

He said there was no indication of any other tumors in the pelvic region, "by sight or feel." There is a cautionary note in that the CEA levels are higher than he would have liked, plus he was obligated to add the caveat that cancer might still remain at the microscopic level. Pathology will report on the tissues in a week or so, but, as he said, "We set up a hard, long, and ambitious approach, and so far, it has all worked out as we had planned."

I am not a doctor, nor do I play one on TV, but to me, he seemed very pleased. In fact, he acted and sounded like an athlete in the locker room after a huge upset victory. I started to tell him how much I appreciated his support, but got choked up and realized I would burst into tears if I tried to continue. It seemed like too much of a cliché to be tolerated, so I tried to convey my feelings with a vague gesture and a series of inarticulate grunts—you know, Guy Talk. No matter how far down the trail to being real you go, there is still a long way to travel.

I spent some time with Mary in her room, a private one, thank God. She was lucid, and spent some time talking with Lori on my cell when she called me for an update. So, bottom line, at this point, things couldn't be better. You want to talk about miracles? We may be looking at one.

But back to the curious title. My old friend Tom Burns loved to tell the story about the farmer who was carrying his prized pig through his apple orchard. Periodically he would raise the pig up to a tree where the pig could nibble on an apple. A passerby saw this eccentric activity, and overcome by curiosity, asked, "Wouldn't it be faster to pick the apples off the tree and let the pig eat them off the ground."

The farmer acknowledged the wisdom of the inquiry, but responded, "What's time to a pig?"

I've often pondered Tom's appreciation of the mutability of time, and whether he ever realized the irony of his delight in that joke, because Tom survived his thirty-ninth birthday by only one day before succumbing to lung cancer. I've thought a lot about Tom these past few weeks. I thought about the injustice of a vital life ripped from this world so prematurely, of the joy he brought to life, of his sparkling intellect. Of the hole he left in my life when he left, and of my utter failure as a friend and fellow human in his final hours.

It was Tom I went to see in the hospital, who turned his skeletal face to me, his eyes unnaturally large and boring into my soul. Because my reflexive greeting was, "How are you doing?" and the very sight of him rendered that question inoperable, I couldn't say anything. His eyes, though I knew cognitively were unnaturally large only because his body was so unthinkably shrunken, served as an accusation. "Is that all you got for me, buddy?" they seemed to say.

I left the hospital that day ashamed, defeated, shrunken as a man. I never saw him again. He died two days later. I vowed never to fail a friend so miserably ever again. I didn't keep that vow, ever. My friend Joe died of cancer. I wasn't there. My friend Bruce died of cancer; I wasn't there. It never got any easier.

Then my friend Mary was diagnosed with cancer, and her prospects were far worse than any of the others. I was there for her. I had no choice, really. I tried to rise to the occasion, through love and devotion. It hasn't been easy. Tonight, when I left the hospital, and even before, when talking with Dr. R., tears were so close to the norm for me that it was hard to fathom. I thanked the surgeon. "You were the first one to give us hope." And he was.

Dr. B., a fine surgeon, by all accounts, though with the bedside manner of an assassin, who did the colonoscopy where Mary's cancer was first discovered, told us in a consultation, after the metastasization was first confirmed, that essentially there was no hope. There would be no surgery. There would be only chemotherapy, and our best strategy was to hope she lasted a year.

Dr. R. gave us hope, and hope is what we have feasted on these past ten months. It was hope strengthened by Mary's marvelous resistance to the deleterious effects of the various treatments she has endured. Her response has been nothing less than miraculous. The love, the affection, the unstinting gestures from friends and family over this past nearly a year were arguably as instrumental as the vast and varied medical procedures she has endured in bringing her to this happy point.

I almost wrote end, but it isn't an end. There is still much work to be done. First Mary has to recover from this latest invasive surgery. She has to learn to deal with her ileostomy. We have another three months of chemotherapy ahead of us, and then another surgery to put her plumbing back together. And always, lurking at the margins, is a turn for the worse.

But still, we are today in a place we never, to be honest, in our wildest dreams, ever thought we would be. Thanks to prayers, from Lutheran, Episcopalian, Catholic and Baptist prayer circles, because Chaldean matrons have lit candles daily, and because, as Karen told me not long ago, she has summoned the Lebanese sisters together for prayer; because Jews have prayed, and even atheists (though Mary maintains atheists can't pray) have sent their thoughts and hopes "up there," Mary is with us, and stronger than ever. Thank you. God bless you.

And finally, a, as I am wont to say, humorous, fact-based anecdote. Last week, the Grosse Pointe chapter of the Herb Society of America had their winter meeting and dinner. This is the one where the husbands are invited. They held it at the Pegasus restaurant in Saint Clair Shores. Over the course of the evening, I watched the women surreptitiously sign a card which they passed. At the end of the evening, they presented it to Mary.

"What's that?" I asked, pretending not to know.

"Oh, just a card," she replied.

"Oh, I wish I had cancer," I said, in a fit of mock-petulance. "So I could get all those cards and gifts."

"I wouldn't wish that on you," she said with feeling. And wait for it, "Because then I would have to take care of you."

I'm so happy I will have that spirit, that wit, and that love around me for a little bit longer. As I told Emily today, "There's no longer a sell-by-date on Mary's life."

January 26, 2011
A Successful Name-Change Operation

The reason I brought Mary home around noon today, was because she didn't think much of my suggestion that she just grab a cab. Which was silly, frankly. I mean every time I've arrived at that hospital, there's been an idling cab out front. But I guess this is the kind of sacrifice I'll have to make for the next few weeks.

Another example: The minute we walked in the door, before I even had the chance to deposit her overnight bag in the bedroom, Mary started boiling an egg. She also made herself a cup of tea. But could she make herself a grilled cheese sandwich? No. I had to do that. As you can see, it's not all fun and games.

We are heartened, and encouraged. At this point, the only cancer in Mary's body, if it is there at all, is microscopic. Of course, that's the way it always starts, so such a phrase is fraught with peril. But that's why she'll have another three months of chemo, so if it is there, maybe we can finally and thoroughly kill it. Only time will tell. In the interim, Mary has healing to go through, plus having to learn the ins and outs, so to speak, of her ileostomy bag.

A strange thing happened in the hospital yesterday. Mary asked for a pain pill because she was feeling minor pain around the incision. (The almost total lack of pain since the surgery is a wonder to both of us, though perhaps, naturally, more so to her). Two hours later she was still waiting. (The story would be a lot more compelling if I could mention at this point that she was screaming in agony. However, that would not be true). Finally, the nurse returned, not with a pill, but with a sincere apology, and a confused look on her face.

Somehow, she explained, Mary had been removed from the system. She was nowhere to be found; she had simply vanished from the computer. As a result, the system wouldn't release the medicine. She promised she was trying to get to the bottom of this. A short while later she returned, this time with more frustration and some urgency. "I don't understand it, but the computer has assigned your bed to a completely different person," she announced.

"Who is it?" we wondered.

"Mary Goodell." Aha, mystery solved. This happened the last time we were at Henry Ford Hospital. Basically, she was admitted as Mary Northcutt and released as Mary Goodell. Truly, a successful name-change operation. Obviously, someone in billing is very traditional, and goes around fixing the records for women who were too "modern" to take their husband's name. Or it was a mix up with the insurance company. We'll get it resolved, one or two phone calls after Blue Cross Blue Shield tells us they won't pay for the operation because there is no one named Mary Northcutt, or Mary Goodell, on my policy. It really doesn't matter who runs health care; if there's a bureaucracy involved, there will be blood-curdling screams.

Anyway, we're both home now. Recovery is on the way. If you want to drop by for a visit, why don't you email me first. That way the phone won't be ringing off the hook. Thanks for all your support, prayers, and love. Now I'm off to make some carrot-ginger soup.

February 25, 2011
You Shouldn't Be Serving Us

Kate and Laura dropped by for a visit one morning. It was two weeks after Mary's surgery. When they arrived, Mary asked if they wanted tea or hot chocolate, and went about preparing things. That's when Kate said, "You shouldn't be serving us."

That's an indication of how well Mary responded to her latest surgery. Her energy was good, the healing process proceeded flawlessly, and her pain was, at worst, manageable. In fact, she never filled her Oxycodone prescription, because she still had most of the bottle from her first surgery. And she still has most of the bottle left. Mary has adapted well to her ileostomy, so much so that the visiting nurse has pretty much limited her services to the occasional phone call.

We managed to achieve our goal of heading up north for Presidents' Day Weekend, and participated fully in the Glen Arbor Chili Cook-Off. It was about thirty degrees, with a light snow falling, as we joined a few hundred others crowded around twenty booths offering everything from traditional three-bean chili to nontraditional Caribbean-style pozole. There is something joyful about standing around with so many people unfazed by cold and snow. It's one of the best things about a northern winter.

#

Earlier that day we had tramped 160 acres of orchards and woodlands with a Realtor as we considered putting in an offer, with an eye to growing grapes and one day opening a winery. Mary has been the prime force behind this pursuit, which is an indication of how well she is feeling, as well as how an experience like this can change your outlook. This is something we have talked about for years, as something we might consider doing someday. With Emily planning to receive her Masters in Viticulture and Oenology in four months, the prospect becomes more real and less theoretical.

The way things stand right now, it looks like the sellers won't agree to our price, so we'll keep looking for the right property at the right price. Meanwhile, Emily will be free to follow the harvest around the world for a couple of years. We'll keep you posted.

By the time we came back Monday morning, fighting ice and snow and heading back to a foot of freshly fallen snow, Mary had started to appear listless and was complaining of discomfort. By Tuesday morning she was emotionally out of sorts. Part of it was the looming resumption of chemotherapy (next Monday), but a larger part was the way she felt. She had started thinking maybe the cancer had come back. This is not an uncommon response, and it makes sense. You've just spent almost a year fighting this disease, and undergone multiple invasive and disfiguring surgeries. Right now, as far as anyone can tell, you're cancer-free, but what if it comes back? This is a killer cancer, and if it comes back, we don't have too many weapons left in our arsenal.

I tried to encourage Mary by reminding her that this was a normal reaction. She acknowledged that truth, but repeated how lousy, and nauseous she was feeling. I mulled that over while preparing her a bowl of soup, and while doing so, I felt a little nauseous myself. And then I realized I had been feeling a little punkish for about a week. I broke that piece of news to

Mary, suggesting maybe we both had some kind of low-grade virus, and she immediately felt better.

Later we learned that there has been a stomach flu going around, so rather than an indication of weakness, the fact that she was only mildly uncomfortable indicated that Mary's immune system is still ticking along as well as ever. It's good not to be sick, even when you are sick.

Speaking of sick, our insurance company seems to have come down with a severe case of incompetence lately. They just can't get anything right. First, there was the $9,000 bill for the last week of Mary's radiation treatment. I got the usual accounting from Blue Cross Blue Shield, only this time, it turned out they weren't covering any of it. There was no explanation, just the bottom line: Your Balance = $8,995. This seemed to require my attention, so I called the customer service number, and waded through the automated help process until I got to speak to a real, live person. Joshua was very friendly, and more than helpful. He was exceedingly patient as he tried to explain why the numbers I was looking at were different than the numbers he was looking at. He helped me understand that BCBS won't pay a claim if the claimant is carrying other insurance.

That seemed reasonable, but wait! I don't have any other insurance. Naturally, he was perplexed. Why would St. Johns Hospital claim I had other insurance if I didn't? Of course, I was a bit perplexed, too. Why would his paperwork show some other insurance company providing coverage when the same paperwork in my hands didn't show it? Joshua was determined to get to the bottom of this. He kept putting me on hold while calling various billing departments at the hospital. He kept getting back to me to inform me that that particular office couldn't pull up the claim, but he was going to try another one.

This went on for about three hours before we agreed that I would just wait until I got the bill from St. Johns, and then we could start it all over again. So that mystery remains unsolved. Then there was the mystery, and the multiple hours on hold, of why BCBS classifies disposable ostomy bags and accessories as Durable Medical Equipment, which our plan doesn't cover. We may have resolved that one.

Then today, Mary came outside where I was shoveling the latest snowfall off the drive (and beautifully, flawlessly sculpting the edges, where they will remain, pristine, until the next person comes over to visit and drives over the edge, ruining my painstaking work—but that's another story), to tell me she had just received "the strangest call from Dr. A.'s office." Dr. A. is the oncologist who is about to administer Mary's latest (and last) three-month-long course of chemo. According to Carrie, in the billing office, Blue Cross says our coverage lapsed as of February 1.

Back to the phones, but first, I needed documentation. I turned to the file for copies of the latest bills. They weren't there. A quick glance at my checkbook showed no checks written for premiums this year. How could I have misplaced not one, but two bills? That's the one bill I pay immediately upon receiving, and have for the past several months. I took my desk apart, looking for the wayward bills. They weren't there. Furthermore, I didn't recall receiving one.

I called, and the automated system assured me that Mary and I were still covered. Then I begged the machine to let me talk to a real live person. It finally did. I told her about the call from Dr. A.'s office. She said, "Well, I don't understand that. You are both covered as of today. Can I do anything else for you?" I explained that I hadn't received a bill this year. She said she didn't understand how that could have happened. I had just confirmed that the address they had for me was correct. But it was clear that I hadn't paid, she agreed. "In fact, your policy is scheduled to be automatically canceled at the end of today."

I managed to pay over the phone, and enrolled in their automatic payment plan, just to be safe. What is really astounding, though, is that she was looking at my account on her computer, which stated that it was scheduled to cancel, but she apparently didn't feel it was worth mentioning it to me. If

I hadn't brought up the subject of the missing bills, she would have let me hang up, and let the policy cancel. Is this incompetence, or is it part of a plan by Blue Cross to jettison a customer who has already cost them far more than she will ever pay back in premiums? An interesting, and disturbing question.

Where this one ends, it's hard to say, but it is frustrating to think that, on top of fighting for her life, Mary is constantly confronting new indignities and roadblocks thrown up by our insurance company.

Mary will be taking different drugs this go-round with chemo, so we once again face a new challenge with uncertainty. She's handled everything else cancer and its treatment has thrown at her, but that doesn't mean this next step will go so well. I kind of feel like the sort of boilerplate disclaimer you see with financial service offerings, "Past performance is no indication of future results." I'll keep you posted.

Thanks again for all your prayers, cards, notes, love, and support.

April 5, 2011
Amazing Grace

Last Sunday, Mary and I went to church, and the service ended with the singing of "Amazing Grace." An old standard, everybody's favorite. While we were singing, I recalled the last time we sang that hymn. It was about a year ago, when we were new to the cancer game, when we were still consumed with decisions which seem laughable now, though they were crucial at the time, such as, "Should we tell people at church?"

I remember we started off strong, but hit the first hurdle somewhere around "saved a wretch like me." I noticed Mary's voice falter, then disappear, about the same time I found it impossible to go on. I glanced over at her. She had tears in her eyes. At least I think they were tears; my vision was a tad blurry, for some crazy reason or another.

The organist finally wheezed out the last notes, none of which had enjoyed our accompaniment. I said to Mary, "We might as well tell them. It's obvious something's going on." So we did, and with each telling, it became easier. The sense of shame washed away. There was no reason to keep it secret;

there was nothing wrong with letting them know. Mary was the center of attention that day, and there was caring, and love, and there were prayers.

#

Last Sunday, owing to quirks in our schedule, was the first in a couple of months in which we attended the service in which the choir sang. Many people were excited to see Mary, as they hadn't seen her in so long. Absence may make the heart grow fonder, but it makes the mind begin to think the worst. So Mary was again the center of attention, and there was much rejoicing.

We're halfway through Mary's final bout of chemotherapy. Just three more cycles, or six weeks to go. Her color remains good, and her energy high. She doesn't have that washed out look that so many cancer patients have, and this is cause for optimism. She has been, in the eyes of her surgeons and oncologists, cancer-free since her surgery in January. Whether that is true or not, only time will tell, but for the time being, we're planning to follow the advice of Dr. R., to "Live well, and live for a long time."

Going back to chemo was depressing, at least for me, as we were surrounded by sick people. One woman was singing the praises of a new surgeon at St. John's. "He's a great liver surgeon," she announced. "When did you have surgery?" another asked. "Back in October. They didn't get all of it, though." "Why not?" "Because they have to leave at least twenty percent."

Then another piped up, "Doctor wants to take my leg, but I said no. I'm eighty-five. That's too old to learn how to get along without a leg." "Well, they took both my boobs," another one said. When we went in, we saw Jeanelle. I wrote about her last summer: "She is a tall, graceful woman with fine white hair, who has carried herself with a quiet dignity. She has also steadily declined physically, so much so that the last time I saw her, I thought we wouldn't be seeing her much longer."

She was still there, looking about twenty years older, and

missing more of her left arm. The thought hit me. Everybody is making human sacrifices to the Cancer Gods. I was going to write that one, but it was too bleak. Even if things are going well for Mary, we remain surrounded by those fighting the good fight. There's no quit in this team, as Wayne Fontes, the old Detroit Lions coach, used to say. They may not have quit, but they're down three touchdowns late in the fourth quarter. Sometimes heart isn't enough.

Along with the no-hopers were the newbies. Another class of parents, spouses, sons or daughters, on their first visit to the lab. They so clearly don't know what to expect, or how to behave. How loudly can we talk? Who can answer our questions? Is this bathroom just for cancer patients, or can I use it, too? It's poignant, seeing their innocence, knowing it won't take long before they're old hands, too. We don't know how their journey will go, because we're planning never to come back here once our course is completed.

Is that true? Who can say? But it was thirteen months ago that Dr. Doom told Mary she probably had a year. Well, we can tear up that game plan. Amazing Grace indeed. But once again, the caveat. That six percent survival rate is based on five years. It's only been one, so we know it can come back, or it might even be there now, lurking microscopically in Mary's bloodstream.

Only time will tell, but we are glad you can share our adventure with us.

May 31, 2011
She's Sick?

After predicting it for two days, Mary came down with a sinus infection, which then developed into a head cold. No doubt this was brought on by all the pollen in the air, which the plants have released with a vengeance every time there has been a break in the rain. I remarked to Mary that this was the first time she's been sick since she got sick, and she agreed.

Which is really amazing when you think about it. This is the first time she's had a cold, the flu, a slight cough, or even the sniffles, in almost 15 months. The whole time she was on chemo, which, among other things, weakens one's immune system, she never caught a cold. I've probably come down with a half dozen colds in that time, but she never caught one. It's really hard to fathom.

Thursday, Mary goes in for her CT Scan at Cottage Hospital. This is the last hurdle she'll face before undergoing her final surgery in July, to reverse her ileostomy. And then we move forward, fearlessly. Of course, if something comes up on the scan, that will change everything. What are the chances something will? Our doctors think they are pretty low. Dr. A. says the only thing that bothers him is Mary's

CEA count, which remains too high.

The CEA, or carcinoembryonic antigen, is a marker which can be used as an indication of the existence of cancer, especially in the large intestine. Normal CEA levels range from 2 to 5. Mary's latest registered 97. Naturally, the doctor would prefer it to go back down to single digits, but he says it may not mean anything. Some people, he maintains, have a naturally high CEA count. Of course, we have no idea what Mary's CEA count was before she was diagnosed with cancer. There was no reason to test for it.

The important thing, is she isn't presenting any other symptoms. Her health has been good (except for this lousy cold), and her energy great. Swing by our house and look at the garden. A lot of work has gone into it again this year, and very little of it was mine. (Though we were out there working together last weekend, when I remembered how last year several of Mary's friends came over and worked her garden for her—that is a memory to be treasured). Then there are the other gardens she helps maintain, and her involvement with various garden groups and other organizations. Most significantly, she looks great. She has never gotten that washed out look characteristic of so many who are dealing with cancer. (Plus, losing that 20 pounds has been a real boost. Mary says it's an effective diet, but she doesn't recommend it.)

So we're just dealing with that one nuisance, that outlier, that high CEA count. But at least we don't have to deal with that question for long, just until Thursday or Friday. Then on Saturday, it's back out to Tucson for a couple of days before flying up to Sacramento to watch Emily receive her Master's Degree in Viticulture and Oenology. Matthew will fly in from New Orleans, so we will be reunited for the first time since his graduation last December. A life in transition, as is the norm.

Thanks for all your prayers and support. Please keep in touch.

June 3, 2011
Nothing to Worry About

Jeanine, Dr. A.'s PA, phoned and left a message today. Mary's CT Scan was "Overall a good one. Everything is stable. There's nothing new for you to worry about." Mary called to get clarification, and finally asked, "Is it safe to say I'm cancer-free for the moment?"

Jeanine replied that she was in stable remission.

That's incredibly good news, tempered only by the fact that when I Googled "Stable remission," I couldn't come up with a good definition. I did find one site which listed the terms oncologists use to describe their patients' status vis-a-vis cancer. Included among them are partial remission, stable disease, and complete remission. Of the three, complete remission is the best one. That's the brass ring of cancer outcomes, the one where there are no signs whatsoever.

Partial remission means tumors have shrunk by fifty percent or more. Stable disease means the cancers are no longer growing, nor are they shrinking. Maybe she used stable remission because there are a couple of nodules on Mary's liver and lungs. They are small, and the same size as in the last CT Scans.

The doctors doubted they were cancerous then, and we can assume, they doubt they are now. But they are still there, which might be why the term is stable remission.

We'll know in a couple weeks exactly what Dr. A., and Dr. R., think of the results, and what terms they might wish to use or make up. (They might have a good laugh if I show them this flourish of medical analysis, but I don't think I'll give them that chance). It's nice to head out on our trip without this hanging over our heads, though. Knowing is always better than not knowing, and doubly so when what you know is good.

While researching oncological terminology, I came upon a meditation called "Just Listening: Narrative and Deep Illness," by Arthur W. Frank. His thoughts on deep illness struck me. That's what Mary has been under for fifteen months, and when one member of the family is, so are the rest. It's true for me, and also for Matthew and Emily, and even our extended family, and all our friends.

"Deep illness may be critical or chronic, immediately life-threatening or long-term," Frank writes. "Levels of functional impairment vary: some of the deeply ill are seriously disabled, in pain, and require intense and constant medical treatment. Others are in stable remission, with their illnesses effectively invisible to strangers and even to work associates. What counts is the person's own perception of illness: illness is 'deep' when perceived as lasting, as affecting virtually all life choices and decisions, and as altering identity. The essence of deep illness is to be always there for the ill person, and the person believes it always will be there. If illness moves temporarily to the background of awareness, that shift is only provisional.

"For as long as one is deeply ill, there is no end in sight. Deep illness is lived in the certainty that it will be permanent and the fear of this permanence."

Notice his use of stable remission. We'll hang onto that diagnosis; we'll work to uproot the deep illness of cancer.

We'll move forward now, eyes fixed on the horizon, where there is a turnstile, and a sign saying, "Thank you for visiting Cancer land. Don't come back soon."

July 11, 2011
A Bump in the Road

That's how we're choosing to deal with this, as a bump in the road. Things were sailing along smoothly, Mary's appointment with Dr. R. ending with laughter, and not quite high fives, but close enough as he laid out the game plan for the ostomy reversal. He also tossed in yet another surgery option, that of removing Mary's mediport, which would well and truly mark the victorious end of her battle. First, she needed another bout with radiology, as they checked to make sure the sutures from the original resection were holding, to make sure there were no leaks, in other words. She passed that with flying colors, naturally.

Then came the phone call from Dr. A.'s office. The results from Mary's latest blood work came back, and this time the news wasn't good. Her CEA levels had risen. The CEA, or carcinoembryonic antigen, as we have learned, isn't totally reliable, which means even if the count is rising that doesn't necessarily mean there is cancer. Conversely, you can have cancer without it affecting your CEA, which is one reason they don't routinely check CEA levels during blood tests.

But the fact of the matter is a rising CEA count is not good. More than anything else, it is discouraging. It feels sort of like that turnstile I mentioned last report, the one next to the "Thank you for visiting Cancer land" sign, needs some oil. It's sticking, and it won't let us through. So tomorrow we offer up some lubrication, our penance taking the form of a Pet Scan. One more ritual in the process which right now is starting to feel never-ending.

Still, following Mary's initial reaction, which was about as discouraged as she has been through this whole adventure, we didn't let it bother us, or slow us down in any way. We went Up North for the Fourth of July, and had the usual good times; good food and good wines with the usual suspects, the cast enhanced this year by the presence of both our kids. Fireworks on the fourth were impressive. We stood at the edge of the lake and watched starbursts from all along the shore. Later, we cooked in the hot tub with Bryan and Rachel, while the show continued. Then, when the red glare of the last of the rockets faded away, nature started her own show, with a brief display of northern lights. What a treat that was.

Since we returned, Mary has been busy preparing for a shower for Kate, one of Emily's friends who's getting married this fall. She wanted to host the reception here, in the form of brunch, outside in the garden. It was a typical Mary production, lavish, stylish, gracefully delivered, and gratefully received. That was Sunday. The Friday before we were in Rochester, attending another wedding. It seems to be a happy season right now, where weddings far outnumber funerals. We want to keep this trend going as long as possible.

Which is why we're calling this a bump in the road, and we head off to Henry Ford Hospital tomorrow expecting the best of results. Send a prayer if you're so inclined. I hope to update you with the good news soon.

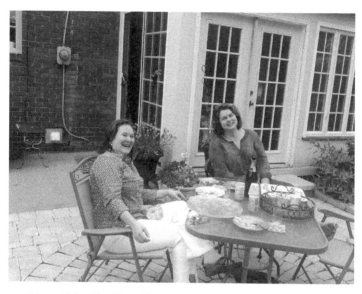

Mary with her friend Josephine Shea, in Grosse Pointe Park, Michigan

July 15, 2011
Or Maybe a Pothole

Well, maybe it's more than a bump in the road. Mary needs four new rims for her car. They're bent, and going faster than 30 miles per hour, it feels like the car is going to shake into little bits and pieces. "Must have been a hell of a pothole," the Belle Tire salesman mused.

Kind of like that. I wasn't sure, but when we got to Dr. R.'s office, all the nurses and office staff seemed extra cheerful to me. Maybe I was projecting, but it felt like false cheer, and the harbinger of bad news. Afterward, Mary said she got the same vibe.

When the doctor prefaces his remarks with the phrase, "I wish I had a happier report," you sort of get the feeling this session isn't going to conclude with high fives. Dr. R. informed us that there seems to be some activity indicative of a tumor along the RFA, or Radiofrequency Ablation scarring in the left lobe of Mary's liver. Also, there are two sites of "hypermetabolic activity" in one of her lungs. The spots in her lungs are very small, and it isn't definitive that they are cancerous, though he feels it is consistent with her "metastatic disease."

What does this mean? We don't exactly know. The balance of the consultation was given over to a lot of "coulds" and "mights" and "maybes," but no clear "we will," beyond his determination that the Henry Ford Tumor Board will reconvene with at least one new participant, a pulmonary expert. Most likely we will be going back to Dr. A.'s office, having to endure the nurses' heartfelt greeting, "Oh, I'm so sorry to see you back."

Mary is frustrated more than anything, reiterating her bewilderment that she should be sick when she feels so good. But she's still strong. When we left the office, she slipped her arm around me and asked, "How do you feel?" Which I thought was performance above and beyond, to say the least.

Bottom line, we're not out of the woods. It isn't going to be as easy as it looked, and probably never was. It is a natural tendency, when things are going well, to believe you're the ones who are going to beat the odds, who are going to lick this thing, once and for all, finally and irrevocably. I can't say it's a mistake to ride that false confidence, because, as all the experts agree, a good attitude is critical to survival. Still, when reality intrudes, and hypermetabolic activity continues, it's difficult to accept it with equanimity.

Now we have to reorient ourselves and understand we're in this for the long haul. We need to get those new rims and watch out where we're going.

Why is This Happening to Me?
August 5, 2011

Asking why is one of those standard stages of the human response to things like cancer. It's in all the books, so we're not exactly covering new ground here. Only, I'm the one asking the question. Things are definitely not going according to plan, and I'm not happy about it. Of course, since I'm not the one with cancer, it's sort of bad form for me to get out front on the whole temper-tantrum-throwing program. Probably better to let Mary take the lead in that department.

Problem is, it might be an awfully long wait as Mary continues in her stoicism. She remains on an even emotional keel, though she is someplace distant from time to time, seemingly taking part in a conversation, but only going through the motions. At times she reminds me of another Mary, who "kept all these things, and pondered them in her heart."

There are things to ponder, such as restarting chemotherapy, a week from Monday. The Tumor Board met at Henry Ford Hospital, and the consensus was that surgery is not an attractive option at this time. Dr. A. discussed various options with us, Mary having pretty much had her fill of oxaliplatin. One of them involved Erbitux, which has been shown to be effective in certain metastatic colorectal tumors. As an indication of how far cancer research has come, and also of how far it has to go, four years ago researchers answered the question of why Erbitux worked well with some patients, but had no effect on others. It turned out it does not work with people who have a mutated form of KRAS, which is a protein that contributes to cellular growth.

As it turns out, Mary's KRAS has mutated, so she is not eligible for that particular treatment. It looks like she'll be going back on Avastin, and along with a new drug, Camptosar, and a couple of the old standards. She'll have chemotherapy for three days every two weeks, each two-week period comprising one cycle. She'll go for at least six cycles, and then we'll reevaluate. Mary says, "Good, I'll have ten days in which I'll be able to travel."

For example, we'll be able to visit Matthew next month down in New Orleans after all. (Matthew, incidentally, told me the other day that it's okay with him if I inform people that he's a hooker in New Orleans. Hooker, for those who insist on knowing, is a position on a Rugby team, said sport Matthew has taken up again after a five-year hiatus).

It really is discouraging to have come so close to getting this done with, only to fall all the way back to the beginning. Mary is going to be one of those returnees to whom the nurses will say, "Oh, I'm so sorry to see you back here." But we will go through with it. It is, as they say, what it is.

But now, for the answer to the titular question. About a week ago, Mary and I had a meeting in Troy, next to the Somerset Collection (for those not from Metro Detroit, the Somerset Collection is a pretentious shopping mall). Emily went with us, and after the meeting, we had lunch at the Capital Grille. It was one of those long, decadent, self-indulgent two-hour lunches. It was the kind of lunch you enjoy when your stockbroker has neglected to inform you that the markets are going to lose more than ten percent of their value in the coming week.

After lunch, Mary and Emily decided some shopping was in order. Having anticipated this development, I had brought a book along. Then I remembered the Tigers were playing a day game, so I went into a place called J. Alexanders, and nursed a glass of wine. Before long a woman joined me at the bar. Her name was Donna, and she was waiting for a friend with whom to share an early dinner. After we chatted for awhile her phone rang, and I listened to her cajole and encourage her friend to join her for dinner.

Donna explained that her friend, John, has just been diagnosed with Stage 4 bladder cancer, and is very discouraged. I mentioned Mary's journey. Then, after Mary and Emily rejoined me, and John joined Donna, we made introductions, and Mary had the chance to encourage John, with her presence and appearance if nothing else, but also, with her optimistic outlook, and her assurance that chemo won't be so bad. I had the feeling it had been awhile since John had last laughed. We left him with a nascent optimism, and the belief that while things might not get better, they could be a whole lot worse.

I guess that's the message we have to take away from this. Things might not get better, though Mary continues to take the attitude that, with treatment, the tumors could just go away. "It could happen," Dr. A. says. "Not likely, but it could happen."

So we'll take it one cycle at a time. Mary still feels well, and looks well, so don't be afraid to call and invite her out for lunch, or for a walk, or a bike ride. That is, if you catch her when she's not traveling.

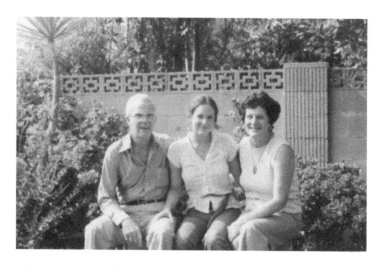

Mary as a teenager with her parents, Val and Nancy Northcutt, in Tucson, Arizona.
—Photographer Unknown

September 16, 2011
Go Ahead and Take That Ride

When I start receiving emails and phone calls and questions during casual conversations asking how Mary is doing, it's an indication that it's time for another update. Usually that means an opportunity to compose another upbeat, cheerful progress report. In a strictly physical sense, that is what this one should be, too.

Mary has completed three cycles of chemotherapy now, and the good news is she's cruising through this round as well or better than she has the previous three courses. Mondays are the monster days, the four-hour sessions which usually knock her out for the rest of the day. Tuesdays and Wednesdays are quite a bit easier. This past week was pretty typical. After chemo on Tuesday, Mary went to get her hair done; then she stopped at church to help prepare for the Rummage Sale. That evening she was off to Belle Isle for the Conservatory fundraiser. It's one of our favorite events each year, though this year I couldn't go. I was sick. Fortunately, Emily was there to go in my stead. Then Wednesday, after chemo, she went to the Windmill Pointe Garden Club 50th Anniversary

Luncheon, came home, put together a program for the Herb Society, and went to the meeting that night.

Last month she went wig shopping, because she was warned that she might lose her hair. Six weeks into the course, it looks like that might have been a waste of money. There's no sign of hair loss yet. So, basically, chemo is just something she does. Kind of like going to the gym, though a lot more expensive, and there are no mirrors or shower facilities on the premises. Apparently, Mary has the perfect constitution for handling chemotherapy. This is fortunate, because we're starting to accept the fact that chemo will probably be a part of her life for as long as she lives.

It is that permanence which is wearing at least one of us down. After coming so close to beating this thing, a little bit of light went out of my world when I realized we weren't done. Those harsh, cruel rules of life do in fact apply to us, too. Sometimes I think I know how a death row prisoner feels. The end is clearly defined, only the exact timing is in doubt. Consider chemo a form of appeals which have to be filed before the judgment is executed. You're just sitting in your cell, waiting for those footsteps in the hallway.

Of course, this is just my perspective. Mary, rather than dwelling on the sentence, is filling her time with the pursuit of dreams and goals, and making plans far, far into the future. We went ahead and bought the land up north and soon will be planting a vineyard. It takes five years before we will have a crop, and probably several years more before our winery will be up and running. That doesn't matter. Mary sits with Emily making plans, designing the winery, the tasting room, and Emily's house overlooking Lake Leelanau. I'll walk into the room where they are making sketches, consulting various magazines and books to get the design exactly right. I'll suggest they are putting the cart before the horse, and they just laugh at me.

No doubt, this is the right way to live, to face the future with a twinkle in your eye, to say, "You think you've got plans for me, but I've got news for you. We're going to do this my way."

Yes, a nice way of looking at things. It beats the nighttime of the soul, the place in which, as bleak as the world looks while lying flat on your back at three in the morning, staring at the ceiling, you know by four you'll look back at three as the good old days. It gets old after awhile. But still we must go on.

Emily wants to make Alsatian wines. It's a good choice for the Northern Michigan climate. We've discovered a great deal about the Riesling grape. It makes wonderfully complex wines, and not just that "dessert wine" for which it is generally scorned in this country. Last summer, while tasting her way through the region, one of the winemakers told her, "We don't drink that sweet stuff, we just ship it to the States." So, what does this have to do with going on? Just this. Next June, Mary wants to rent a house in Alsace to celebrate our thirtieth anniversary. I'm doing the research. I'll make the plans, and we'll expect to have a great time. We hope to have some friends join us for part of the time.

It's much better to view your future with excitement rather than fear. While you stand in line to board the roller coaster, you hear the screams of the other riders, and the rumble and clatter of the cars. The tension mounts. It is frightening, yet thrilling, too. As the line gets shorter and the time to board gets closer, you don't think about all the things that might go wrong; you try to figure out how to time it so you can sit in the front of the first car. All the better to get the maximum thrill from the ride.

We can all learn from Mary's response to her cancer, me most of all. Thanks for your support and prayers and gestures of kindness and friendship. They are valued more than you will ever know.

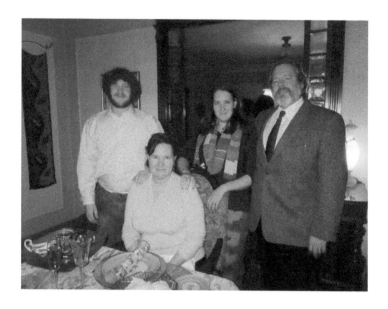

Posing at the table lavishly set for Christmas or Thanksgiving was a semiannual tradition.

—Photographer Unknown

October 26, 2011
Sometimes it Just Happens Like That

Yeah, she actually said that. Mrs. Jones, a Customer Service Supervisor for Blue Cross/Blue Shield of Michigan, actually said, "Sometimes it just happens like that." That was in response to my question, repeated for the eighteenth time in the previous two hours, "Last year after May, when your statements read 'The patient's copayment requirement has been met,' we weren't charged another copayment for the rest of the calendar year, and this year, after February, your statements read, 'The patient's copayment requirement has been met,' we weren't charged another copayment until August, when the statements started to read, 'The out-of-network copayment of $11,600 has not been met.' What is the out-of-network copayment, and why did it suddenly appear?"

It seems a simple enough question, one which a customer service representative ought to be able to answer, and if not her, then certainly her supervisor. Instead, she says things like "We changed our computer system," or "That's not what it says," and "Nothing has changed, that's the way it's always been." When that approach gets tired, she can always fall back on, "Sometimes it Just Happens Like That." Which is why after I finish this update I'm driving downtown to the Blue Cross/Blue Shield building, files in hand, to finally get some answers. I guess you could call it my own personal Occupy Blue Cross movement.

#

Last spring, when I mentioned that BCBS had changed to an electronic billing system but had neglected to inform some of their customers, which meant we almost lost our coverage, our friend Sara, who played my role for a couple of years while her fiancé fought the good fight (and is currently winning), told me to get used to it, that I would be spending a lot of time fighting with them in the future. I didn't want to believe it was true, but I now don't know what else to think. Actually, the most disturbing thing of all about this is when I quote Sara's prediction to the BCBS Customer Service people, they don't even bother denying it.

We've been going around this week telling people Mary was on her last cycle of the latest course of chemo, and after that, we'll test and see if there's been any progress. Yesterday we learned from Dr. A. that cycles last two rounds of chemo, not one, so we are in fact only half way through this latest six-cycle course. This wasn't the first time Dr. A. contradicted himself, but it was the first time I started to doubt him.

The good news is Mary is handling the chemo as well as ever. Every other Monday, when she has her long day, she's pretty much wiped out, and tends to sleep most of the day. But she has very little nausea, and her hair isn't falling out. One day out of 14, that's not too bad.

Another three months of this, on the other hand, is discouraging. It does get old. All the charm of the place has long since dissipated. The jokes have grown stale. There's nothing new left to learn about the process, and the sight of people pitching forward off their chairs in the waiting room is not one you want to get used to. But, we're back at it, or still in it, and in this case, the old cliche is true. It does beat the alternative.

Just a little while ago Dr. A.'s office called to give Mary the results from her latest blood test. Her CEA levels, while still high, have fallen by half, from 139 to 69. This is movement in the right direction. It indicates that the chemo is having an effect. So we'll have another CT Scan in a couple of weeks, and who knows, maybe by the 27th we'll have something to be truly thankful for.

Thanks again for all your love and kindness, and prayers, and support.

November 23, 2011
Happy Thanksgiving

When the world shifts you learn to look at life in a different way. The little things that once caused so much frustration, the way someone cuts you off in traffic, or the cashier in a grocery store who would have to pick up the pace a bit to earn the title of automaton, somehow they don't matter as much anymore. You learn to appreciate friends, and to value those who show you that they really are. You learn to be awestruck by their many random kindnesses, the little gestures, the extension of a hand, or the offer of a shoulder to cry on.

Sunsets, though they never passed unremarked, become little miracles, the better to be savored. The clarity of late afternoon light, cutting through the haze to set a maple tree ablaze, to cast the autumnal brown of the oak tree vivid against the slate gray sky, you learn to treasure those moments. One came a few days ago, when Mary called me up from my office to "see the light," and worthy it was of wonder.

The sight of the children across the street, acting out the storybook of their young lives, reminding us so much of our own children at that age, becomes a gift to be treasured. We stand behind our windows and spy on them, and want to give them the gift of eternal youth. Though we know, of course, that it is a false hope, a faulty dream. We learn to value the embrace of the church, the comfort of ritual, and the miracle of prayer.

There is so much to be thankful for. The kids are both home for Thanksgiving, and Mary will be cooking it again. That is a tradition we definitely want to preserve for years to come. We can be thankful that we are eight months and counting past the date our first doctor told us would be the end of counting. We can be thankful that today Mary told me not to bother going with her to chemo, because she planned to go shopping afterwards, for supplies for Thanksgiving, and for the Tree Trimming party we'll host this Saturday.

I did meet her at the doctor's office in the afternoon, to review the Cat Scan she had last Thursday. The good news is her liver is stable. There are no new lesions or growths, and what abnormalities there are, are "related to surgery." There is no sign of cancer in Mary's liver, lymph nodes, colon, or rectum. Unfortunately, the report also says "Several pulmonary nodules in the right lung have enlarged since January 2011, consistent with progressive metastatic disease."

Dr. A. asks, "How large are the nodules?" The report doesn't say. It says they've grown since January, but what have they done since July? That is the latest urgent question we need to answer, which is why Mary is going to get a Pet Scan next week. We can compare that to the one she had in July, and decide where to go from there.

Basically, it's bad the nodules have grown since January, but it will be good if they have shrunk since she began her latest course of chemotherapy. Sometimes it seems like nothing more than a game, a cruel game refereed by a sadistic fate, who dangles the promise of release, only to push the goal line a little bit further down the field. Or, to put it another way, Mary is Charlie Brown, the football is remission, and cancer's wearing Lucy's dress.

So, we have something else to look forward to, another test, another exam, another consultation. But we do have things to be thankful for, not least, I suppose, is the fact that when I visited Frankisha at the Blue Cross Blue Shield walk-in Customer Service office today, she remembered me, remembered Mary, and remembered our case. Sadly, she asked, "Didn't someone call you?" Apparently the person she spoke to who promised to resolve the issue called back to say she couldn't do it. Frankisha called someone else while I was there, who said she'd take care of it. It is a process. How kind of the insurance company to provide these distractions, to take my mind off the battle with cancer.

Mary continues to run on all cylinders. She sleeps a bit more than usual, though she maintains she's always been a napper. And that's true. She continues to make plans for the winery, and I continue to dream of remission. Here's wishing you, one and all, a Happy Thanksgiving. Don't forget to savor the miracle of life, and the gifts of beauty God offers us each day.

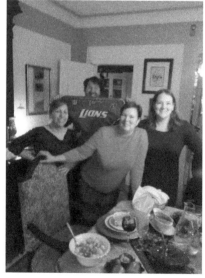

In 2015 Matthew married, and Nora became part of our family

December 8, 2011
It's a Wonderful Life

Every year, when the press of the holiday season starts to wear, and the rampant consumerism rankles even more than it usually does, at the point just before I start crying, or throwing things, I'll sit down and watch "It's a Wonderful Life." It's the one time in the year when I allow myself to be emotionally manipulated. I go into it knowing my heart will be tugged, and tears will form in the corners of my eyes. More than knowing it, I expect it, and the year I don't get that little catch in the back of the throat is the year I'll have to start seriously thinking about hanging up the stirrups.

The preceding, in journalism speak, is known as "burying the lede," because attempting to make the title choice pop-culturally relevant is not the real point of this update. No, the real point is to report on Mary's visit with Dr. A. As you may recall, her recent CT scan results showed nodules in her lungs had increased in size since January, and were "consistent with metastatic disease." The doctor noted that the fact that the nodules had grown since January gave no indication whether the chemotherapy we began in August was working. He prescribed a Pet Scan, and the results were the reason for the visit.

According to the Pet scan, "tiny right upper lung nodules are seen without abnormal activity. These are too small to characterize on PET images." Or, to quote Dr. A., "Mary is in complete remission."

"It's always good to get good news heading into the holidays," was Mary's reaction, along with, "I knew I was feeling too good to be sick." My own reaction was a little more muted, perhaps skeptical would be a better term. I'm still sitting here waiting for the other shoe to drop, for fate to stick the knife in just as soon as I let down my guard. Or maybe it's just shame at having been so defeated since the middle of last summer when we found out we weren't done after all.

For now, we are, although we'll have another month or two of chemo. Dr. A. says Mary isn't cured, and the cancer most likely will come back, but as long as she is handling it, we might as well finish the course. The further we knock it down, the longer her remission might be. Makes sense to me.

After all, there's nothing sporting about cancer. There are no Marquis of Queensbury rules, no Lady Byng Trophies. With cancer, you do want to hit him when he's down. Rabbit punch? Just fine. Blindside hit? No problem. What the heck, we'll even taunt cancer. We'll run him out of town on a rail. Cancer will never eat lunch in Mary's body again. There's no law against bullying cancer, and when speaking to cancer, hate speech is not just accepted, it is mandatory.

I wonder now how long before our lives get back to normal, whatever that was or will be again. Or maybe they never will. Maybe we will never take another sunset, or sunrise, or friendship, or family member for granted. Maybe we will continue to approach each Christmas as if it might be our last together. Or perhaps, in time, life will subside, and the commonplace becomes ordinary becomes unremarkable, and we will forget what a difference a day makes.

Maybe, in time, we will forget these crucial lessons

forged in the furnace of mortality. And maybe, just in case we do lapse into complacency, that won't be such a bad thing after all.

We will never forget the kindness, support, prayers, and love from so many friends, new, old, and rediscovered. This has been the most amazing gift of all, and definitely one which won't be taken for granted. As I type these words, I can feel the tension finally slipping away, and I am starting to believe it's okay to believe.

Merry Christmas.

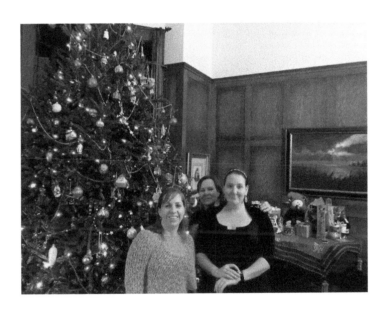

January 11, 2012
Good-bye to All That

Mary had a busy week this week. Monday was her last really long chemo day. She couldn't go home and nap though, because she had a lot of work to do planning a brunch for 15 set for Tuesday morning. Tuesday morning came, and Mary and Emily were making quiches and baking brie, and setting out tables and chairs. Okay, I was setting out tables and chairs. I pitched in where I could until the guests arrived. (I find that I become more like a cat with each passing year–when people start coming through the door, I sneak down to the basement and hide until they're gone).

After the brunch ladies left, we went back to chemo, then over to the produce market so Mary could buy herbs with which to make bouquets *garnie* for the Herb Society's Annual Dinner on Wednesday night. Then, after chemo yesterday, she met Kelly, Josephine, Kate, and Emily at the Dirty Dog Jazz Café for lunch. The HSA dinner at Dylan's followed that night, and, as Mary said to me this morning, "What a wonderful night of sleep that was."

So we're done with chemo. For the time being, Mary says. Forever, I correct her. We're done forever. Her cancer is in remission, and it won't be coming back. You can trust me on this one, because I'm a doctor. Well, not really, but let's just pretend. We have a full winter, spring, and summer planned, because you should always strike while the iron is hot, while both the spirit and flesh remain willing. We are gifted with today, but who knows about tomorrow, my medical pretension aside.

The other day, Mary received a call from a friend at church who wondered if she could speak to another friend who had just been diagnosed with Stage 4 colorectal cancer. Mary was happy to do so, and called and gave her as much encouragement as she could. There is something about hearing what is going to happen from someone who has been there, someone whose voice is strong and cheerful, who has been to the precipice, stepped back and decided you might as well live.

It was a gift Mary has been given, to have this kind of knowledge, and a gift she willingly shared, to shine a light on the trail on which her friend has just embarked. It's bizarre, really, that at any time there are some five million people in this country fighting cancer, yet when you get that diagnosis, you feel so alone. The world continues to spin, but somehow you aren't part of its normal functioning. Everyone looks different to you, and you know, in time, they will look at you differently as well.

Yesterday counts for nothing, and tomorrow is a mystery beyond utterance. You have no one but yourself, and maybe your spouse and your children, though really, even if they're there, their understanding is only on the most shallow of levels. They really can't know what you are going through, what you are thinking, and what streams of consciousness flow through your brain. It is such a gift at a time like that to be able to hear from someone exactly what is going to happen, when and why, and to make the offer, "Feel free to call me anytime, for anything."

That is a gift Mary has been given, and a gift she now is able to give.

May 10, 2012
We're Fighting Again

At first, I was hesitant to use this title, because I thought it might convey the wrong message, that we were back fighting cancer again, instead of the one I wanted to send, which was after nearly six months of remission, things had gotten to be so normal that we had returned to doing the sort of things normal couples do, like having little spats from time to time. Cancer was no longer a day-to-day companion, a parrot on Mary's shoulder, squawking, "Awwwk! Thar she grows." If anything, cancer had receded to the point of being something of an inside joke.

Then during a routine appointment with Dr. A. yesterday, Mary mentioned having a little colorectal discomfort. He agreed she should make an appointment with Dr. R. In the meantime, he took some blood to run some tests. He called today, saying he'd considered waiting until we got back from our big anniversary trip to Alsace next month, but decided it would better to call now, to let us know that Mary's CEA count has gone up, from 69 to 100.

This doesn't automatically mean that the cancer is back,

as we have noted previously and repeatedly that the test is not foolproof, that the counts can fluctuate dramatically with each test, and even though normal CEA counts should be below five, they aren't always, and we don't know what Mary's normal count was since they were never counted until after she got sick. On the other hand, it isn't the most positive sign, either.

Our plan now is to go ahead with our trip—I just paid the non-refundable balance on the house we're renting in Riquewihr today–and expect the best. Then sometime in July, Mary will have another CT Scan, and then we shall see what we shall see. Probably the worst case would be that Mary would have to undergo another round of chemotherapy. Dr. A. mentioned during Mary's visit yesterday that the woman in the next room had been given a diagnosis similar to Mary's ten years ago, which means, though it can be a real nuisance, this sort of cancer isn't an automatic death sentence. People can and do live with it, for a very long time.

I'll let you know what happens next just as soon as we know it.

August 6, 2012
Damn Hubris

In my last update, I mentioned that Mary's CEA count had risen, which suggested that her cancer had returned. It wasn't definite, and according to all our doctors and advisors, not worth changing our travel plans. So we didn't. We had a marvelous time, visiting wineries and staying in quaint German and Alsatian inns. We caught up with our English friends, Malcolm and Caroline and Nigel and Sabine. Emily was with us, and Matthew joined us for four days.

There were times, especially after our friends had returned home, when Mary basically spent a day flat on her back; when Emily and I shared our fears that Mary's cancer was back. I viewed with increasing trepidation a raven which seemed to lift off from a roadside meadow whenever I rounded a curve in our rental car, or we emerged from a stand of trees on another hike. I'm not given to superstition, but the symbolism grew irksome.

As our trip continued though, through Champagne and into Paris, Mary seemed stronger every day. Maybe the pace of the visit had been just too much. Maybe we all needed a day to unwind, and Mary was just more susceptible to the nap. After we returned home, her energy continued to be high, and we never really slowed down.

Bryan and Rachel's wedding was at the end of June, and we hosted Ron and Shelley from Montreal. There were cancer survivors from Toronto and Boston, and when we joined them for an impromptu swim party at Mark and Molly's on the Saturday before the wedding, it was a case of A Cavalcade of Scars, all worn triumphantly by those emigres from Cancer Land.

After the wedding, there was the little matter of a colonoscopy before we headed up to Glen Lake for the Fourth of July. The test revealed no hint of cancer, and Mary's blood tests were good. Plus, our friend Paul told us the rule of oncological thumb regarding CEA counts was "plus or minus thirty," which was how much Mary's count had jumped. So on to the cottage, where Chuck and Ruth Anne joined us.

Then we threw ourselves into the vineyard property, clearing a road through the woods and starting to work on a stone wall at the entrance. Meanwhile, Mary headed out to Tucson to get her mother's house ready for sale. We'd rented it for a year-and-a-half, but now it was time to test the market again. But first, a little TLC was in order to refreshen it. Mary was there for ten days, up at dawn each day, and working through. Her energy was tremendous, so much so that my inability to accompany her to her Pet Scan on the 24th was barely a blip on the radar. Mary Beth stepped up, and they spent a pleasant afternoon together afterwards.

I wasn't really all that concerned about the test, telling someone I couldn't imagine how it could possibly be positive—I hadn't seen a raven in weeks. Mary was feeling too good, was too energetic, and we had a full summer planned working on the vineyard property. Such is the case with hubris.

We didn't even bother inquiring about the results until we returned home last Monday. Mary called Dr. R.'s office, and the secretary said he had sent her a letter, and to follow up with her oncologist. "That doesn't sound very good," Mary said.

We pawed through the pile of accumulated mail until we found the letter. Among other things it said, "There are multiple nodules throughout both lungs." The largest of them showed "intense FDG activity." FDG stands for fluorodeoxyglucose, which is the sugar most commonly used during a Pet Scan. The sugar goes wherever cells are most actively growing; the brighter the spots, the more intense the activity. The report said the "remaining nodules throughout both lungs are mildly increased in size from comparison and demonstrate range of FDG activity from none through moderate."

There is also some indication that there may be some activity in the liver, though based on my reading, it is not definitive. But the lungs are pretty straightforward. Of course, it's important to remember that Mary doesn't have lung cancer, or liver cancer. She has colorectal cancer which has spread to those organs. Ironically, there is no indication whatsoever of any active cancer cells in the colorectal region.

We met with Dr. A. today and began to chart a response to this latest news. He has an interesting manner about him, treating cancer as a routine matter. He always cites someone he's just finished seeing who has been at this twice as long as Mary has, and is doing fine. It's all very reassuring.

Next Monday, Mary has an appointment to get a new mediport installed. She had her last one removed in the spring. That was back when we had this thing well and truly licked and were only looking forward. Now, we're back into it. Mary's a little disappointed as it will be another scar, but as Emily told her while we were in Europe when Mary noticed that her blouse had slipped to reveal a scar, "That's a war wound, not a blemish."

And when Mary resumes chemotherapy on August 20th, it will be a strategic repositioning of troops and neither a defeat nor a retreat. If all goes well, we'll be at this for four months, which means she'll be off chemo in time to host our annual Christmas Party. In the meantime, I'll be spending less time up north. There are a number of encroaching trees I was planning to cut down which just might have received a reprieve. At least for awhile. Few things in life are certain, but two of them are as soon as Mary finishes this round of chemo she's going to resume beating the drums for that Australia trip, and those trees coming down, sooner or later.

In the meantime, polish off those prayer beads and get back to work. We'll be in touch.

October 12, 2012
The Thrill is Gone

This past Monday, while I was sitting in the chemo lab with Mary, the man in the chair to my right kept remarking how slowly the day seemed to be moving. He knew all the nurses by name and showed complete familiarity with the system and scene. He wasn't acting like one of those people who blame the entire world for their having contracted cancer, and are sworn to make everybody else's life as miserable as their own. He was merely stating a fact as he saw it. Mary was sleeping, and I was drowsing, and so I agreed with him that something did seem off.

"Well, I've been doing this for twelve years," he said, blankly, a statement of fact, an assessment of the reality of his world. I knew instantly what he meant, and understood why his day was moving so slowly. He was hooked up to the bags and was stuck there until they finished dripping. There was nothing interesting there. The thrill had long since passed for him. This was just the way things were. This was how he was consigned to live his life. I got that in an instant, because I have been reeling with dealing with the same blunt reality. Even though I'm not hooked up to the bags, I might as well be because this is the brutal fact of my life as well as Mary's.

The thrill may well be gone, but at least the process gives us, or him and Mary at least, a fighting chance. So I said, "It beats the alternative," as much for my benefit as his. He gave me a look after I said that. It wasn't hostile. It wasn't argumentative. If anything, it was probably closer to pitying. As if to say, you really think that, eh? Give it time, my friend. This is as good as it gets.

Already halfway down that road, I wasn't necessarily surprised by the sentiment though it did seem to violate the unwritten rule of always pretending that a day at the chemo lab was fun, fun, fun. Maybe he just recognized a fellow traveler.

Ever since Dr. A. pronounced Mary cancer to be "incurable" back in July, this is the way the world has rolled with me. The thrill is gone. There is no longer any there there. This is just the way our life will be. The doctor was confident that Mary could continue to live a good, quality life for many, many years. She tolerates chemo well, and the cocktail of drugs has been effective in the past, and there's no reason to think it won't be in the future. In fact, Mary got a call today from the doctor's office informing her of the results of Tuesday's blood test. Her CEA count has dropped precipitously, from 160 when she started this latest round of chemo, to 100.

No doubt you all recall that CEA stands for carcinoembryonic antigen, and that the normal count is somewhere between two and five. Which means Mary isn't out of the woods just yet, but the chemo seems to be doing its job again, and we have every reason to believe that by December her cancer will be back in remission.

That's our expectation, because we are much too busy to allow this cancer thing to get in the way. Mary has been moving pretty much nonstop since she resumed treatments.

She claims it is affecting her more than it did last time, though Emily and I both know this isn't true. Last fall, every other Monday, which was her long day then and is still now, Mary would come home and would be asleep before I could finish making her soup. And the soup was Top Ramen, so it's not like making it was a long, drawn-out affair. This time, she hasn't even napped on Mondays. She just keeps going.

This was actually rather fortunate since Mary had agreed to allow our house to be included on a tour for a group called Questers during their recent convention. A couple hundred people passed through the house. In addition to cleaning furiously, and getting a lot of plastering and painting done, Mary also decided she wanted to serve refreshments for the tourists. Which she did. A massive job performed as a matter of course.

This weekend she is hosting an Alsatian Feast for some of the people who built the Equipment Storage Facility on our vineyard property Up North, along with some local vintners and some close friends. We'll serve Choucroute Garnie and Backeoffe, and Tartes Flambees, washed down with local Dry Rieslings, in the newly finished building. Not quite a stone table overlooking acre after rolling acre of vineyard, which is the setting for feasts in every winery-themed romantic comedy ever filmed, but it's a start.

Mary has a couple of meetings scheduled for later next week, and a Herb Society Tea on Saturday. After that, she's driving to Grand Rapids, where she will meet me at the conclusion of my bicycle trip from Traverse City. It's just a short one this year, only 160 miles, but circumstances having prevented me from taking one at all last year, it will be a relief. We look forward to a nice dinner, and a pleasant evening at the Amway Grand Hotel, then it's back home for another round of chemo. After that, a week on the Outer Banks with our friend Lori, then we descend into the maelstrom of holiday obligations and events.

And so we beat on, boats against the current—hmm, I rather like that. Kind of catchy, don't you think? We are rich in friendships and blessed with the warmth of faith and hope. Thanks for your support. Keep Mary in your prayers, and give her a call from time to time. Again, she's handling chemo well and is always happy to go out.

December 31, 2012
Auld Lang Syne

It's New Year's Eve, and we have big plans. Sit around, maybe watch a movie, possibly a bowl game (I think there's a new one on tonight, the Tidy Bowl—but I could be wrong). Maybe around midnight we'll open a bottle of champagne, and switch channels to see if there's any coverage of the "D Drop." It's the third year the City will commemorate the closing of a year with its own downtown celebration.

It's also the third year that we will have celebrated New Year's Eve since we got the dreadful news. It's the third calendar we've torn from the wall since we read those horrific words, "six percent survival rate." We sat numb. We wept. We prayed. We moved on. We lived. And now, another year has passed, and Mary is feeling as fine as ever. Dr. A. says she is handling her chemotherapy so well, he wants her to keep going. So she'll start her fourth month of three treatments every two weeks. Her markers continue to drop, and there is no liver activity whatsoever. These are all good things. We won't know what effect the treatments have had on the tumors in her lungs until we do another Cat Scan, probably toward the end of January. But the important thing is, we are alive, and we continue to live.

Mary got a dog for Christmas, a Black Scottie named Mason McDuff. We spend hours just laughing together, watching the dog tear up the house, pulling tablecloths and lamps to the floor, chewing up Mary's mother's fine china. Oh, the fun we will have! (More good news—three New Years later, and I still have my sense of sarcasm).

So many friends have seen their cancer return over the course of the last year. Bruce, Chris, Dave, Diane. For others, like Bonnie, the diagnosis is new; the journey is just beginning. For still others, the diagnosis is the same; the cancer remains. Some of them should be dead by now, but they refuse to cooperate. They just keep plugging away.

I ran into an acquaintance at a Holiday Party whose remission ended in May, around the same time Mary's did. Quite a change from last year's party, when he was exultant at his remission, and I was sure that Mary was finally, well and truly cured. He wasn't happy when he learned it had returned. We talked about this. And about his feelings, his mood, his loss of hope, and subsequent resignation. And then we talked some more. And some more. And I realized what a gift I've been given, to be able to stand there and listen to someone pour out his soul on a subject most people can't wait to avoid. Oh sure, you want to ask "How's it going?" and maybe get a thumbnail report on status and prospects, but you don't want the unabridged version.

I know. I used to be that guy. In fact, I was the guy who was afraid even to ask the question. Now things are different. For Mary and for me. Because, as PJ put it a couple summers ago, I "have Mary's cancer, too." And it's not bad. We both move forward. We both take hope from the flipping of another calendar page. We'll drink a toast to the year gone by, and to tomorrow, and then on January 7th we'll meet the new year, same as the old year, and I'll drive Mary to chemo. And then I'll drive her home, and we'll start to undecorate the Christmas tree, and friends will call her and invite her to lunch and go on walks and we will go on. We will continue to look death in the eye, and laugh at death when it finally blinks, again.

Happy New Year.

March 7, 2013
Something in Leather, Perhaps?

Last Sunday, somewhere around noon, we passed the Third Anniversary of Mary's diagnosis. Yes, it's been three years since Doctor Doom gave Mary a year, and offered "chemotherapy and hope it works." The surprising thing is, the anniversary happened without either of us realizing it. Actually, that's happened occasionally with our wedding anniversary, too. As a general rule, if both parties forget it, there is no harm done.

Mary had another CT Scan last month, and the radiologist who read the scan, our friend Paul who read it for a second opinion, and Dr. A., Mary's oncologist, all agree that the current regimen is working. She still has cancer, primarily in her lungs, and as everybody seems to delight in reminding her, it will probably be with her forever, and is incurable. But the chemo is knocking the tumors down. They started small and are getting smaller. This is a good thing.

The other good thing is Mary continues to tolerate chemo in remarkable ways. She just finished her thirteenth biweekly course, and after she left the lab, she went straight to the

Garden Club Luncheon, for which she had baked a Key Lime Pie and Gingerbread before going off to chemo. I remain amazed at Mary's resilience. I am also stunned by how seamlessly Mary's cancer has been woven into the fabric of our lives.

I still recall the chill, the terror and the utter foreboding of the first diagnosis. When we sat on the couch and stared blankly at the wall. When she apologized for not getting checked out sooner, and I apologized for not realizing that she was sick. When we decided right then and there not to apologize anymore. That is how we started our journey, and this is how far we've come. There will be many more milestones before we are done.

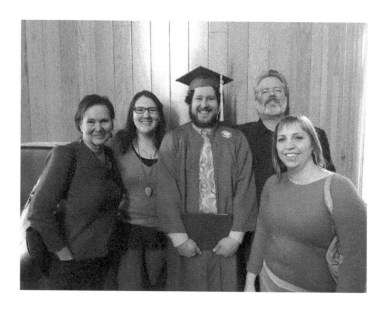

As our family's vineyard developed, Matthew pursued a degree in viticulture from Michigan State University under the innovative Vesta program, to compliment Emily's Masters in viticulture and Enology from UC Davis.

May 16, 2013
A Willful Retreat

I'm writing this in an empty house. No dog, no chickens, no people. It's quiet, and gloriously empty. One of the reasons the emptiness feels so good is because it is volitional emptiness. The house is empty, because Mary has made her annual Mother's Day retreat to Glen Lake. She took the dog and the chickens, and life is good. Volitional departure is so much better than that arbitrary form which is so cruel, so remorseless, and inevitable; though it will be a retreat we all must one day take, most of feel, as the Nubian slave did when he told Maximus, "But not yet, not yet."

Yet it will come, and often not at a time of our choosing. A young friend lies in critical condition after an auto accident last Saturday. One moment his life is unfolding before him, the next, the subject has changed, for him, his family, and his friends. It can be so arbitrary when it comes, whether its taking is sudden or steady. It is the background noise to our existence, the soundtrack to our personal movie. Whether we think of it or not, it is there. What we do with our time while it lies at bay is what determines whether or not we have lived successfully.

Maybe, as Gerald and Sara Murphy were wont to say, living well is the best revenge. But don't wait for life to sink its claws into you, exact anticipatory vengeance. Live well now, and all the rest will follow.

Mary was late for her Mother's Day retreat, because the first three days of the week were occupied with chemotherapy. When she finished on Wednesday, she was finished indefinitely. Her CEA count, though still elevated, is dropping. Her liver enzymes are perfect, Dr. A. says. Her health is solid, her energy is good, and so, after nine long, boring months, her latest bout with chemo has come to an end. We will have a busy, active summer, flying to Minneapolis for a wedding, driving to Toronto to see friends and then flying to the Gaspe Peninsula, which is located, well, one hopes the pilot will know.

We'll spend much of the summer up north, putting down roots and digging up trees, watching our adventure unfold, living as well as we possibly can. If you're around this summer, try to make plans to drop in for a picnic in the vineyard.

As for the future, only time will tell. The cancer is still lurking in Mary's body, hiding out behind the occasional cell. How long it will stay hidden is anybody's guess. We left the doctor's office with the unspoken expectation that we'll be back, maybe by the end of summer, but who knows? It's not written in stone. There's no law that says it can't stay away, this time. But we might as well live as if it's gone, gone for good. If it's only on vacation, no problem. So are we.

July 13, 2013
Why Me?

Thursday we went to Dr. A.'s office for a routine checkup. We discussed our strategy going forward. In a word, our strategy consists of doing nothing, which proves that, when it comes to cancer, the old cliché rings true. No news really is good news.

Dr. A. says Mary continues to be asymptomatic. All her markers are where they're supposed to be, except for that pesky CEA count, which has ticked up again. But the CEA is notoriously fickle. The rule of thumb in the cancer world is CEA +/-30. So since Mary's count went up about thirty points, we'll disregard it. Unless Thursday's blood test shows another rise, in which case we'll schedule another Pet Scan.

In the meantime, we continue in our summer of contentment. After we left the doctor's office, I suggested a late lunch on the water. We went to Brownie's on a pleasant, not too warm day. There were just enough clouds to hold off the sun's merciless rays while we sat on the deck and watched a flotilla of boats, large, small and gargantuan, float by.

Then last night we were on a boat ourselves, with John and Diane and Bryan and Rachel. They took us across the lake and down the river, to Bayview, where we sat dockside dining al fresco and listening to soft jazz under the sunset-turning-starlit sky, on a night which couldn't have been more perfect if we'd personally drawn up the plans.

Today, we head back Up North where Emily will put us to work in the vineyard, and the following week we're off to Canada for a week of visiting friends and relaxing on the shore of the St. Lawrence River.

So the perfect summer continues, a time of contentment marred only by occasional loss, regret, and for Mary, a curious reversal of that standard cancer victim's plaint. "Why me?" she wonders, though in this case, it's not the self-pitying question why she's been selected for this challenge. Rather, the inquiry, posed with a sense of wonder, is why am I still here?

We've seen too many since Mary was diagnosed, whom she has comforted, counseled, and encouraged, who have finished their race ahead of her. "Why me? Is this even real? Why do I feel so good? Why have I cheated the odds, and is it right or even safe to wonder?" Because one of the worst things about cancer is the way like time's swift arrow it ever lingers at your back. It's never over, but sometimes it goes away for awhile.

And sometimes others go away forever. Mary's sense of survivor's guilt was heightened when our friend Bonnie finished her fight. It came quickly, almost without warning, and took her just as fast. She was always so bright and lively, so alive, that just knowing her made you feel like a better person. Cheerful and upbeat, almost to the end, the world was a lesser place when she left it. She left Mary wondering, "Why me?"

Maybe the lesson, if there must be a lesson, is to never lose sight of the wonders that comprise our existence. Each sunset, each newborn day, every minute and every mile, should be met with wonder, should be greeted with the question, why me? Why have I been granted this gift of life?

October 1, 2013
A Way of Life

No doubt most people have already figured it out. We haven't been reticent in our confidence that sooner or later Mary was going back to chemo. Her CEA count rose steadily all summer. Now, we've been over this several times. We all know that it isn't the most reliable count, that the numbers can vary with each test, and that the rule of thumb is CEA +/- 30. But when it goes up all the time, that's not a good sign.

And so it was as we reached the end our summer of fun and friends and hard labor in the vineyard, of travel to new places, making new friends and reconnecting with the old, as the days shortened so too did our sense of reprieve diminish. Last month we went back to Dr. A.'s office where we learned Mary's CEA count was up to 250, the highest it's been since she was first diagnosed. The CT Scan was ordered. I told Mary to study hard for this one. She just gave me one of those looks, the one that means "You can't study for a CT Scan, you idiot." I'm sure she meant it affectionately though.

We got the results last Thursday, the day after we returned from Tucson, a working vacation to spruce up

Mary's mom's house in another bid to sell it, but also time spent with Martha and Becky, Mary's oldest friends, and with the Babbs, our former neighbors. Frank has published a novel, so it was kind of a treat to have dinner and compare our publishers and our sales experiences.

The test results weren't good. The tumors in Mary's lungs are growing again, at an increased rate, and the activity in her liver, which we were always able to dismiss as likely ongoing post-operative healing activity, has finally defined itself as a tumor. The good news is no new colorectal activity. It is important to stress here that Mary doesn't have lung or liver cancer, just colorectal cancer in those organs. The other good news is we can resume the same treatment we ended last May. Mary has a proven tolerance to this treatment, and more important, she has responded well to this particular cocktail of poisons.

So there's no reason not to expect a return to stable remission a few months down the road, and maybe another long, fun-filled summer vacation. Mary remains upbeat and symptom-free, her major complaint is the hassle of scheduling her chemo sessions around her book club, herb society, and garden club meetings. Not to mention the holidays which are rapidly approaching. When should we have the tree trimming party? And the big Christmas Party? And can you believe it? She's supposed to have chemo Christmas week! What a nuisance.

I suggest to her that maybe she's got her priorities wrong. That she should focus more on the treatments and less on the ancillary activities. She gives me one of those looks again. And she's probably right.

Last update, I mentioned the survivor's guilt she's been feeling, as people who have been stricken after her, whom she has counseled and consoled, have lost their fight too soon.

Then there are the others, the old hands like Bruce (whom we were privileged to visit this summer) and Tom, who are in the same boat as Mary. Their cancer will never go away, but they continue to live because that's just what you do. It struck me, thinking of them, and of Mary too, that cancer isn't just a way of dying, it is also a way of life.

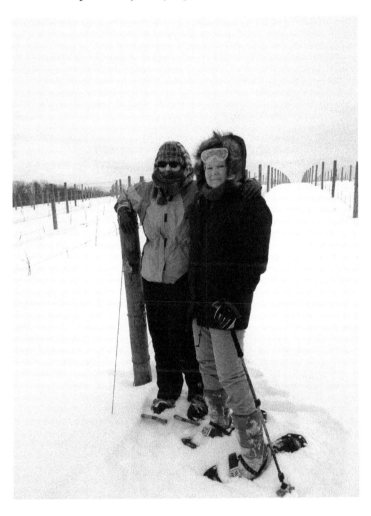

Emily and Mary inspecting first year vines in the winter of 2013-14 at our vineyard in Leelanau County, Michigan. Producing and selling our wine was a dream Mary fought hard to realize. Every glass we pour is in her memory.

December 19, 2013
In the Tall Weeds

It seems cancer has been springing up like weeds around us of late. Two invitees to our Christmas Party said they would attend if they weren't knocked out from chemo. In one case, that was the first we heard they were sick. It comes up quickly, and sometimes strikes you down completely, as happened to a friend's brother. Just ten days between diagnosis and death. He never had a chance. His family was still in the information-management phase, the one where you try to decide who needs to know and how soon, before you figure out that it really doesn't matter. Everybody is going to know, because life as you once knew it has ended.

Another long-term cancer survivor was telling me about an article he read about changing attitudes toward cancer treatment, and how to keep people alive. I asked, "It's just a matter of quality of life then?"

"No it's a matter of quantity of life," he stressed, meaning the longer you stay alive, the better your chances that they might have figured out how to beat the particular strain you're fighting. Maybe this revolutionary new approach called immunotherapy, which trains the body's immune system to attack cancer cells, will actually be the magical cure some think it might be. It will take years of research and experimentation to know for sure. So, yes, quantity does matter.

A fresh perspective. I'm not sure if I could do it. I don't think I'm strong enough to put up with all the pain, the stress, and the inconvenience; the trading of quality for quantity. Then again, I don't have to. Because this story isn't about me; it's about Mary. She doesn't seem to have those issues. She just trudges along the path God carved out for her. She successfully negotiated a successful Christmas Week program, so she won't be wearing the pump on Christmas Day.

Her counts are going down, and her markers remain quiescent. Dr. A. is pleased, and so are we. Our insurance was canceled, but we found a new plan which will allow her to keep her doctors. So Mary is pleased. Our premiums went up by fifty percent, so Blue Cross Blue Shield is pleased. My new novel is being published tomorrow, so maybe I can pay for those premiums. Everybody seems to be happy. There's snow on the ground and lights on the tree, presents under and everybody coming home. We'll go Up North until the New Year and start at the chemo lab just three months shy of four years of survival.

We stand here, on the threshold of the new year, surrounded by tall weeds as friends right and left get laid low. We can be there to encourage them, to help them back to their feet, and to assure them, well most of them, that there is life after diagnosis; maybe we can add a corollary to Gerald Murphy's Law. How about, "Living long is the best revenge?"

We'll see how that one goes. In the meantime, Merry Christmas, everybody.

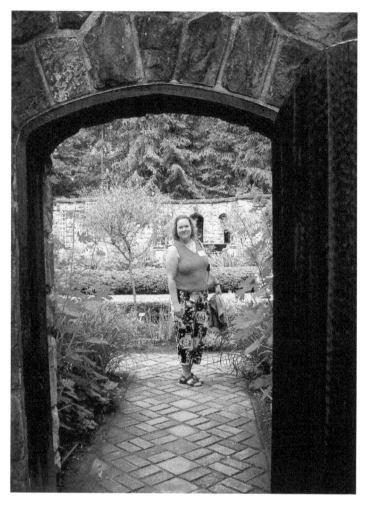

Never more at home than in a garden, Mary was a perennial attendee at the Herb Society of America's Annual Meeting.

— Photographer Unknown

March 6, 2014
The Uninvited Guest

We celebrated a birthday this week, but we didn't throw a party. Even if we had, the guest of honor would not have been invited. Not that it matters. He would have shown up anyway. He's always there, but he's never welcome. He doesn't need an invitation, because he already lives in your house. In fact, he lives inside us, literally and figuratively.

The guest is cancer and the birthday was his fourth. It was four years ago this past Monday that Mary was first diagnosed with Stage 4 Colorectal cancer, and next week will mark four years since the doctor said she had about a year to live. So this definitely falls into the category of good news.

Mary has been in chemotherapy since October, and will probably be there through the end of April. After that, perhaps another summer off. She had a CT scan last month which indicated that the tumors in her lungs and liver have stopped growing, and in fact are shrinking, and in some cases breaking up. These are all good things. The only negative is her CEA count, which remained high, and while it fluctuates, its trajectory is ever higher.

Which means there really isn't any new news. She still has cancer, and probably always will, but so far we have a regimen we can live with. She continues to handle chemo extraordinarily well. She has yet to get that washed-out "I've got cancer" pallor to her skin. And, as she jokes, she seems to be the only person in the world who gains weight while on chemo.

The challenge will come if the cancer adapts to the drugs she's receiving, or she can no longer tolerate the treatment. That will constitute the next step in our journey. Fortunately, for the time being, there are no indications that this will happen any time soon. So we will beat on, looking forward to a few months off, with a number of weddings to attend, and a conference in California which will enable us to visit my folks, and of course, hours of labor in the vineyard Up North. It's hard to think about summer when there are still three feet of snow on the ground, but it will be here soon enough, and soon enough ended as well, and before we know it there will be a fifth birthday, and maybe when we hit number five, we will have a party.

May 9, 2014
Summer School

I had planned to entitle this update "School's Out For Summer," as we approached a second annual summer off for good behavior, a stage where Mary's tumors having been beaten down to the point of near invisibility, and her cancer having reentered the stage of stable remission, she could take three or four months off. It evoked a sense of normalcy reminiscent of our youth, when each year we were released from the stuffy old school room, bursting into the open to relish the freedoms of summer.

That was the plan, and there was no reason to think it wouldn't have played out that way. Mary had her CT scan, and we waited for the results. A call from Dr. A.'s office that there had been only minimal changes since the last scan. Mary made some joke about how those minimal changes had better not be for the worse. We could joke about that sort of thing, because we had this cancer thing down to a science. It was just routine, and we had made a lot of plans for the summer.

Then came the doctor's visit, and the news that the change was in fact for the worse. The tumors were larger, which meant the chemo was no longer working. It was a reminder from cancer about who is in fact in charge. It isn't Mary. It isn't us, it isn't Dr. A., or nurses, or surgeons. It is cancer. Cancer is like a very good pitcher who changes speeds and angles, always keeping the batter off balance and off his game. Cancer lets you get used to one program, and then it changes the rules. Cancer never lets you rest.

Cancer is the most passive-aggressive of diseases.

And now cancer has messed up our summer. Mary will still take some time off, until probably mid-July, after another CT scan to see how rapidly the tumors are growing, and while Dr. A. comes up with another chemotherapy cocktail. Then we'll start up again, and see how it goes. It's a tough process, going from first thinking we'd licked this thing, only to learn that wasn't true. Then we reached a point where we had it under control. Mary was living with cancer, and living well. Now, we're entering a new phase, one where cancer, after taking a couple years off, is starting to flex its muscles again.

Just to be clear, the prognosis is not dire. There are other chemo options, and some new drugs that have come on the market, and if those don't work there are always clinical studies. In fact, there was an article in today's Wall Street Journal discussing a new procedure which shows a lot of promise. Even if nothing works, which is to say if Mary strikes out in every at bat, the tumors are growing so slowly that Mary has plenty of time left to enjoy the vineyard, gardening, travel, sunsets by the lake, living well, and getting her revenge.

So that's where we stand. To borrow from Winston Churchill, "This is not the end, this is not even the beginning of the end; but it is, perhaps, the end of the beginning." Now, Churchill was referring to a different war, one which many might say was more significant than the personal battle Mary is fighting, and they would be right, from the perspective of history. But though we are just two little people piling up a hill of beans, this war is the big one. This battle is the only one that counts.

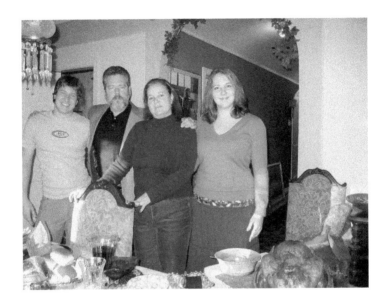

July 14, 2014
Welcome to the New World

Mary had an appointment with Dr. A. today, where we learned the results of her latest CT Scan. Tumors in both lungs and the left lobe of her liver continue to grow. The largest one, in her left lung, can be measured in centimeters now, and not millimeters, and they seem to have grown by twenty-five to fifty percent since her last scan. If that weren't enough, Mary admitted for the first time to feeling some discomfort. She said maybe it was just sore muscles, but she hasn't really been doing anything physical. (Actually, she has been working in the garden, so maybe she did strain a muscle. Time will answer that question).

Obviously, this wasn't a good report, though Dr. A. still considers the growth to be slow. The next big test comes when Mary resumes treatment, probably next week. She'll be going on a new regimen, involving a pill called Xeloda, or Capecitabine. She'll take the pill every day for three weeks, and have one week off. In addition, she'll get Avastin by infusion every other Monday. There's some question whether our insurance company will pay for this particular drug, and how much our copay will be if they do, but that's okay. I haven't really had much chance to talk to the nice BCBS Customer Service people since our insurance got canceled last December. It will be nice to resume old friendships.

Speaking of which, we did just that last month when we took advantage of Mary's "summer break" to spend some time in California. She and Emily attended the Herb Society of America's Annual Meeting, along with my mother, whom Mary invited to join them. My Dad and I got to go golfing, which actually turned out to be fun (amazing what a different game it is when you aren't consistently hitting balls into the woods).

We got to spend time with old friends and, miraculously, revive a friendship I had feared lost forever. We spent two nights in San Francisco, toured Napa a couple of times and had one amazing, memorable dinner which we will be talking about for years to come. When we came back, we headed up to Glen Lake for the Fourth of July. Emily's friends Matt and Laura joined Bryan and Rachel, John and Peachy, for a good and proper celebration.

We've been working hard on the vineyard property, putting in rock and water gardens and developing a landscaping plan. Emily is getting intimately involved with the viticultural aspects of the operation, which is what she has wanted to do. Matthew is pitching in when he can. He and Nora went off to Italy to attend a wedding and maybe plan one of their own. Before they left, they bought a house in Traverse City. Emily is about to move into a condo there, as soon as they finish building it.

I think in some ways this is a case of Mary tidying up her kids' affairs, just in case things head south. I don't know for sure, but it feels that way. We like the shape of her new chemo schedule as it will give us a little more freedom for being Up North and traveling to Vermont and Montreal, two big events in the offing for August and September. Of course, the key to the treatment is its effectiveness and not its convenience. One reason we're doing this one is to avoid Oxiliplatin, because that caused neuropathy in Mary's feet, and we don't want that.

It this works, great. We can do that. If not, then we'll enter the horse-trading stage, where Mary will have to decide how much sacrificing she wants to do to keep on living. In a way, it's the sort of negotiations all of us do each day as we give up a little bit more of our dreams in exchange for the gifts of the day to day which constitute our existence. With cancer things are different. The sacrifices are greater, the consequences more severe, and the negotiator is always happy to just walk away from the table. In other words, cancer is Putin, and we're the Ukrainian army.

For the time being, we move ahead. Pray that this regimen works, and that Mary continues to enjoy good health. Well, good health except for that obnoxious thing called cancer.

September 9, 2014
On the Road Again

Before Mary started her new chemo regimen in July, her CEA count, which for the past four years had fluctuated in a range between 60 and 130, and had never before tested above 238, had soared to 1046. I had missed that doctor's visit, being Up North trying to help out with the vineyard. When Mary told me that piece of news, it brought me to a very dark place. But, for most of us, most of the time, the light comes back on eventually.

Mary's new routine is a lot more user-friendly, involving just one half-hour infusion of Avastin every three weeks. She is also taking a new drug, called Xeloda, in pill form twice a day for two weeks, and then has one week off. It has allowed us to keep to a busy summer schedule. Happily, in the early going especially, Mary wasn't feeling any side effects at all. In fact, she began to doubt the treatment was even very effective.

So in a sense, it was almost a relief when side effects did appear. Her hands had turned a brilliant red, looking, according to the marketing mythology, as though she had washed dishes without using Ivory Liquid. Worse, her feet became very sensitive. It felt, she said, as if her soles were covered with blisters. Walking became a painful experience. It also, Mary being Mary, became an excuse to go shoe shopping.

After consulting with Dr. A. they agreed to cut the dosage from six pills a day to four, and to take a second week off. Which means Mary returned to chemo yesterday, on her sixtieth birthday. She wore a pair of glasses in the shape of the number 60, and the nurses got together and sang "Happy Birthday" to her. Some of the other patients joined it. A sweet moment. Even sweeter, Dr. A. says Mary's CEA count has plummeted more than 300 points, and her latest x rays indicate that the tumors in her lungs have gotten smaller. Her liver markers are solid, and all her other counts are right where they should be.

He ushered us out of his office with the phrase, "You're on the road to remission."

So, very good news. Of course, to keep things in perspective, 745 is still extremely high for a CEA count which is normally 2.5–5; the tumors may be smaller, but they're still visible to the naked eye; and though being on the road to remission is a very fine ride, we've gone down that road before, only to hit a detour before we reached our destination. So we can temper our hope with realism.

Mary has always been so skilled at compartmentalizing her cancer, accepting it, dealing with it, fighting it, yet not letting it affect her life. It was the same this summer, spending time up north, hosting friends from both near and far. We went to Burlington, Vermont for a wedding, and chose to drive, staying in Oswego, NY, then driving through Adirondack State Park before taking a ferry from Port Kent to Burlington. A perfect three days in Vermont before a leisurely drive home, the only damper being Mary's tender feet.

Since then it's been one event after another, culminating tomorrow in a trip to Montreal. The Montreal Racquet Club is putting on a five-day commemoration of its 125th anniversary. I told Mary it was officially called the MRC 125th Anniversary and Mary Northcutt Sixtieth Birthday Extravaganza. I suspect she doesn't believe that's true, but she's going along with it to humor me.

Mary's hanging in there, living life to the fullest. We attended a Garden Party fundraiser for the Belle Isle Conservancy this evening, and I just stood back and watched all the affection flood her way. Same with her birthday party last Saturday. When you are surrounded by friends, and love, maybe that is the best way to treat cancer. It certainly helps you understand what makes life worth living.

October 10, 2014
Remission–Again

Last time I checked in, you may recall, Mary was on a new medicine, called Xeloda, which she took in pill form, along with one infusion of Avastin every three weeks. The treatment was working, but the side effects included blistering hands and feet which made walking excruciatingly painful. Dr. A. reduced the dosage by a third. This had the desired result of greatly diminishing the side effects, but it left a serious question begging. Would Xeloda work at the lower dosage?

This week we visited the doctor and got our answer. Yes. Mary's CEA count dropped by another 300 points, and is down to 460, which is still high, but is definitely going in the right direction. Dr. A. explained there are three kinds of remission: stable remission, where the cancer has stopped growing; remission, where the cancer isn't growing, and in fact the tumors are shrinking; and total remission, in which there is no evidence of cancer at all.

We're at the midpoint, just plain old remission. Cancer isn't active, the tumors are shrinking, and if all goes well in a couple of months, they will be too small to read with an x-ray.

Maybe Mary will have another CT Scan at that time, and then she can take some time off for the holidays.

We've been busy, juggling work in the vineyard Up North with chemo appointments. I've been cutting down trees. Mary and Emily dealt with Sophia, the last of our chickens. Maintaining her became untenable since Emily has moved into a condo in Traverse City, and Matt and Nora have bought a house there. Emily resolved to do the deed herself, and with Mary's assistance, killed, plucked and cleaned the bird, and cooked it in Riesling. Circle of life indeed.

We've been busy, traveling to Montreal, and hosting friends from Williamsburg, VA, and Wisconsin. Next month, Mary's going to Los Angeles for a few days, to see old friends and catch up. Maybe she will be able to tell them she's done with chemo for the foreseeable future. That would be a nice development as she heads toward her fifth anniversary.

January 6, 2015
A Journey, Not a Destination

We headed Up North the day after Christmas, and stayed there until January 2nd. On New Year's Eve, we went to a new restaurant in downtown Traverse City called The Franklin and participated in their loud, raucous, and typically exuberant New Year's celebration. We got to see the cherry drop, and the fireworks fly, and hug and kiss perfect strangers while shouting, well, you get the idea.

I spent much of the week describing various activities as "A Journey, Not a Destination." Losing weight, recovering from the cold Emily and I both came down with four days before Christmas, chopping wood, they were all journeys, not destinations. Maybe I hit the theme a tad too often, because both Mary and Emily began greeting my observation with a particularly pained expression. They do that sometimes, and I always seem to know when and how to get under their skin. Call it a gift.

The holidays were busy, packed with visits and gatherings and parties, parties, parties. It's a form of economic indicator, I believe. As the economy improves more people want to share their good fortune, or at least support the joys of the season. And there were plenty of reasons to be joyful. Mary's continuing good health, Matt and Nora planning their wedding, Emily enjoying her condo and working hard on the winery project, having a family business and starting to get the feeling we'll all be around for a long time to enjoy it.

Even though Mary's CEA count had risen at her previous blood test, to 590, up considerably from 510, but still down dramatically from the 1290 it reached before starting this particular course, Dr. A. maintained she is in remission. She feels good, and is presenting no symptoms.

Yesterday we had an appointment, and learned her CEA count had dropped to 550. Now, to keep things in perspective, that's still twice what her count was when she started her first course of chemotherapy back in 2010, and 250 times a normal count. But she feels good, and we expect the next CT Scan will show that her tumors continue to diminish.

I've been doing some reading about advances being made in immunotherapy. Intrigued, and compelled by the CEA uptick, I created an online profile for Mary and discovered there are some sixty-six clinical trials for which she might qualify, many of which are in the Detroit area.

I discussed it with our friend Paul, the radiation oncologist, and he thought it was a good idea. One thing he explained was we didn't have to move to Houston or New York to get into a clinical trial at MD Anderson or Sloan Kettering. We would just go for three or four days while they run tests, and then they would set up a program that can be administered here in Detroit.

That's an encouraging sign, though Dr. A. told us yesterday that we probably wouldn't qualify for any of the tests right now. The reason? They want active cancer cells so they can better gauge the effectiveness of the trial. Maybe one day, he told us, we can pursue that, but not now, because we don't need to.

One thing we do know is we are just two months away from an amazing milestone. It will be five years since Mary was first diagnosed. Since we sat there, gobsmacked, looking at the bleak prognosis, the chemotherapy and hope for the best, the maybe you'll get lucky and can have surgery, the horrific, unblinking, black-and-white numbers stating that the chance of her being alive in five years was a paltry six percent.

That may be what the experts said (it has since gone up to twelve percent, incidentally, which shows what great progress is being made in fighting this disease), but it's starting to look more and more like we beat those odds. And if we can beat those odds, who knows what other odds we can tackle?

It's a new year, one filled with hope and plenty of plans for the future. One thing we know for certain as we move into 2015 is surviving cancer is both a journey and a destination.

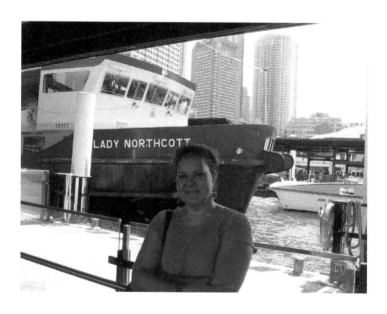

March 4, 2015
Preaching to the Choir

Last Sunday, as church was letting out, one of the members, having noticed me sitting by myself, approached, and asked with some concern how Mary was doing. "She's fine," I replied, pointing at the choir loft where she sat enrobed.

"That's a wonderful reason to be sitting alone," she exclaimed. And it was. It certainly beat a number of alternatives for sitting alone, as others are learning now.

A month or so ago our friend Tom surrendered after an eighteen-year fight with cancer. How courageously he fought was summed up best by an oncologist friend who said Tom's cancer should have taken him after just six months. So he added more than seventeen years to the balance sheet.

Tom was the one who told me Mary didn't care about six percent odds, or twenty percent. "There are only two numbers she cares about," he told me in no uncertain terms. "Zero or one hundred percent."

One of Tom's sons mentioned that rule during his funeral. It was an amazing ceremony, filled with outpourings of love. Everyone there realized no matter how well they knew Tom, with the exception of a lucky few, they only knew a small part of the complete man.

It is rare indeed to hear people say after a funeral that they envied the man whose passing they just commemorated. In death as in life, Tom epitomized the philosophy that living well is the best revenge.

Cancer never stops giving. It is forever reaching out, welcoming new friends with open arms. Shortly after losing Tom we learned another friend has been diagnosed. His dispensation: another eight years. Well, we shall see.

Mary and I are getting ever more excited as Matthew's wedding day approaches. Mary is elbow deep in preparations, arranging for the centerpieces, buying flowers for the arrangements. Family and friends will be coming in from all over the country, and even from abroad. It should be a fine celebration of love and joy.

Mary's in Lansing this week, with Emily, attending the Michigan Grape and Wine Conference. It's been another disastrous winter, with record low temperatures. It has been so severe we may not have any harvest whatsoever. As a result, we've put off building the tasting room for another year.

Mary wasn't thrilled with that idea, "and I think you know why." I did, and do, but it can't be helped. I told her she'll just have to plan on sticking around a little while longer.

After the wedding, we have some decisions to make regarding Mary's treatment. Her current regimen, while not an utter failure, seems to be fighting a rear-guard action against the disease. Call it an orderly retreat if you will. While the tumors appear to be growing at an exceedingly slow rate, the number of tumors isn't increasing.

However, her CEA count soared in the last test. It had been drifting around in the 500 hundred range, up or down thirty or forty points, which meant it was basically stable. But now it's back up to 1,000. You can do all the rationalizing you want, but that is still ominous.

We'll sit down with Dr. A. the week after the wedding

and discuss our options. We might go back to one of the previous regimens. Sometimes they can regain effectiveness as the cancer continues to change. There remains, too, the exciting world of clinical trials. This would involve some travel, and a new realm of experience.

We'll keep you informed. In the meantime, we are barreling down the home stretch of the first leg of our journey, with our eyes focused on the future, and with a renewed commitment to live just as well, and as long, as we can.

March 17, 2015
A Joyful Noise

It started heading south when Matthew reached the front of the room and turned to face the assembled guests. I stood and gave him a hug. His eyes showed he was moved, and I felt the waterworks begin. I sat down and said to Mary, "That was a mistake."

Mary always reminds me to take a handkerchief with me when I go to a wedding, because one never knows when a lady might be overcome with emotion. Still wedded to the belief that I am a cold-hearted, stoical rock of a human being, not given to outbursts of emotion, I will, unless reminded, neglect to bring one along.

As I did for Matthew's wedding. When I remarked on this oversight, Mary mentioned she had a handkerchief, "with flowers on it," if I wanted to use that. I declined, and wiped the tears away with my hand, and regained my composure before it was time to participate in the parents' reading.

I wasn't alone. A great many of the guests were equally tearful, leading me later to wonder how it could be so joyful when so many people were crying. It was such a wonderful time, seeing all of Matt and Nora's friends, from all over the world, gathering to share in their special day. And so many of our friends were there as well, as well as my parents and my brother and his family.

When our friends thanked us for inviting them, I tried to make it clear that I had nothing to do with the invitation list. Violating the basic rule that, once you find yourself in a hole you should stop digging, I continued plugging away at my explanation. It wasn't that I didn't want them there, or wouldn't have invited them if I had had the choice, but to me it seemed it would be more special for them to know they were at the wedding, because the bride and groom wanted them there.

Amidst the festivities was Mary, celebrating her fifth-year cancer anniversary, a once-unlikely always improbable guest at her own celebration. Not just the mother of the groom, Mary took it upon herself to do all the floral arrangements for the wedding and reception. Granted, she had help, including Emily, whose condo rapidly took on the aroma and appearance of a florist shop--a very small florist shop. A florist shop that had outgrown its space.

Emily's friend Barb, whose wedding we attended a couple of years ago in St. Paul, was also a great help. They got the arrangements done on Friday, then Mary was up before dawn on Saturday to deliver the arrangements to the Opera House. I kept waiting for her to collapse, to surrender to fatigue. I expected we'd make an early night of it. I certainly didn't expect to be dancing with her following dinner, nor did I expect her dance card to be filled for the rest of the night.

I also didn't plan on removing all the decorations from the Opera House at the end of the night, but those were the rules, and we complied, Mary plugging away with the rest of us. We returned to the hotel well past midnight, but made it up to greet the newlyweds at brunch the next day.

So here we are, five years and one day from my first entry, and still, we take things one day at a time. Still, we move forward with a death sentence hanging over us. The other day I decided this is an approximation of a death row inmate—though, of course, Mary has committed no crime—the sentence weighing over his head, the execution stayed for years through legal maneuvers, appeals, and pleas. Except in our case, there is no governor to commute the sentence. We've been convicted, and she will have to face the masked man on the gallows. We know this. We've accepted this. The one thing we don't know is when this is going to happen.

The amazing thing is, as long as Mary is around there is no one to remind me of her fate. She continues blithely along, refusing to even nod at time's winged chariot. Life is for the living, and by God, she chooses to be among them, and if I want to tag along, I'm welcome, and so are you.

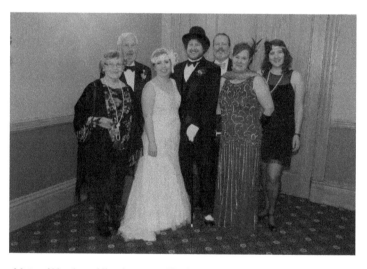

Matt and Nora's wedding theme was The Great Gatsby, and everybody dressed for the part. From left, Martha and Malcolm Goodell, the bride, the groom, Michael, Mary and Emily

—Photographer Unknown

June 22, 2015
A Hill of Beans

Mary had a small crisis at chemo today. Just the usual Oxaliplatin blues, but this time a bit more severe. Tightness in her chest and down her arms drew a cluster of nurses and the PA to her side. Her temperature rose, and her blood pressure spiked, and the experts were scurrying around, doing what they could do to stabilize her, which they did. They cut off the Oxaliplatin and infused her with meds until she was able to finish the treatment.

What made this one different was the large number of newbies in for their first visit to the chemo lab. I could feel their eyes on us, and their trepidation, their wondering "Is this what it's going to be like?'

Unlike other influxes of newbies, neither of us felt much like showing them the ropes. We kind of left them hanging, knowing they too would, if they were lucky, become old hands, watching other rookies come in and feel their way.

Looking at them, reading their doubts and their fears, I felt like Humphrey Bogart in "Casablanca," at the Cafe Americain, responding to the desperate young Bulgarian bride with a stern, "Everybody has problems, maybe yours will work out."

The thing is, unlike Bogie, cancer rarely has a change of heart. We keep going through the motions, keeping our appointments, taking those tests, all the while pretty certain cancer isn't going to come into the casino, put his finger on the roulette wheel, and rescue us from a visit to an oleaginous Captain Renault.

Cancer's going to kill Major Strasser all right, but he won't let Ilsa Lund get on that plane with Victor Laszlo. Cancer's going to get the girl in the end. He always does.

Come to think of it, cancer got Bogie, too.

As I write this the sky pulses with lightning. I watch the flashes through the window wells leading to my basement office, and I think that is highly appropriate. Sometimes it just gets you that way.

But that's my status report. Though Mary continues to suffer through this particular regimen, as she has through none of the others, losing one and sometimes two days of every fortnight, she is, otherwise continuing to do well. Even though her bad numbers continue to climb, they are, as Dr. A. says, climbing more slowly, and her tumors seem to be relatively stable. In a couple of weeks, she'll go in for another CT Scan. While making the arrangements, I remarked to myself how effortless it is to deal with hospitals and receptionists now. It used to be such an ordeal, but now I know who to call and what to say and can answer their questions reflexively. We've come so far.

We'll know more after the scan. Then we'll decide what to do next. There are still some clinical trials out there, and other medical systems to explore, but how long we'll stick with this particular regimen, I don't know. I realized the other day that next month will mark a full year that Mary has been receiving chemo without a break.

It's amazing she can handle it as well as she has, even though each week seems to be worse than the last one. When she isn't flat on her back every other Monday, she remains remarkably busy, hosting dinners and meetings, installing new gardens and tending the established ones, while developing the landscaping at the vineyard property Up North.

Her energy level is amazing, except when it isn't. She naps frequently, has developed a nagging cough, but happily, she doesn't have any pain. And so we beat on. Every day a new beginning, another challenge, another milestone. We always try to keep in mind that our problems don't amount to a hill of beans in this crazy world.

We have a full summer of work ahead of us, between treatments, and look forward to Bryan and Rachel and Bruce and Nancy joining us for the Fourth. Friends from California will be visiting in August, and Malcolm and Caroline (and maybe Nigel and Sabena) will travel from England to help with the harvest in October. Maybe we'll see you around, either here or there, for a light supper or a lunch date, or, if you find yourself in Leelanau County this summer, for a lakeside visit.

August 12, 2015
Houston, We Have a Problem

It's been a month-and-a-half since my last update which ended, as you may recall, with Rick and Louie walking across a fog-shrouded runway in Casablanca, speculating about the breadth and scope of their nascent friendship. A bit of a cliffhanger, that one, promising enlightenment following Mary's latest CT Scan. A bit of a tease, since more than a month has passed since she had it.

So to bring you up to date. Mary hasn't had chemo since the end of June, and she feels, all things considered, great. The bad news is the reason she stopped taking chemo. It wasn't working. All the bad counts keep getting worse, and her tumors are getting bigger. She has developed a painful sounding wracking cough which she insists is allergy related, but deep inside even Mary has to acknowledge it's due to the tumors in her lungs.

Well, these are the days we didn't exactly sign up for, but we accept in due course as the terms of the contract are never clearly spelled out when you enter the arrangement called life. Here we face the challenges of the next step in our adventure, this one involving a trip to MD Anderson, to undergo a battery of tests in the hopes that there might be some promising study looking for subjects just like Mary.

We leave next Tuesday, and will be gone until the 26th of August. Mary's first-day schedule has the feel of the first day at college, with orientation and registration, followed by a series of exams. They even call their complex a campus, just in case the analogy wasn't getting through.

As everybody knows, there is no more desirable place on the planet than Houston in mid-August. Temperatures in the 90's, with humidity to match. We wanted to stay in the hotel across the street from MD Anderson, connected by an enclosed walkway. Unfortunately, they were fully booked. We're in a hotel .4 miles away. I told Mary we would drive to the hospital, "Because I don't know if you'll be in any condition to walk that far." She laughed and said she was sure I was the one who wouldn't be in any kind of condition.

She was right. I have no doubt upon walking out the door of Houston Hobby Airport I will wilt like Blanche Dubois (means white wood) once Stanley Kowalski unleashed his macho charm.

We have come to this point, because there is nothing left in the standard oncological bag of tricks. There are no viable surgeries. There is nothing but hope and resiliency, which Mary has in spades. Me, I just stagger along and try not to wake up in the middle of the night.

One positive, we discovered while filling out the lengthy New Patient Profile online, is the Mary is in remarkably good health for someone who has basically had incurable cancer for five years. We think some researcher might find her status appealing as a subject of one of his or her trials. That's the hope, anyway.

We'll let you know how things go. Maybe I'll even file a report from Houston.

In other news, we experienced the Megastorm of 2015 at Glen Lake on August 2nd. We saw our sixty-foot-tall Blue Spruce snap off and fall to the ground, followed by our screens blowing in and the trees beginning to dance. It was then we decided to run to the basement. (It was then our dog, Mason, decided to play keep away). We thought we were victims until we learned what had happened in Glen Arbor, on the other side of the lake. Nature's power is awesome.

The next day we went to the vineyard and learned that, though we were spared the winds, we had had three-and-a-half inches of rain in an hour. That was enough to wash out our roads, but we were spared structural damage. Then, we learned that the rain was mixed with hail, and that took out almost our entire grape harvest.

Truly, this has been our Summer of Discontent.

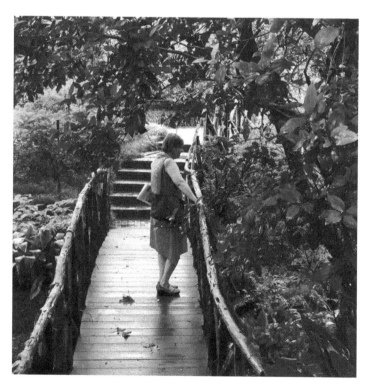

A contemplative moment at the Ima Hogg House in Houston, Texas.

August 28, 2015
Houston on the Seine

Of all the surprises to come out of our visit to Houston, the number of very good French restaurants has to rank among the top. We expected barbecue, Tex-Mex, and Vietnamese restaurants, and there were plenty of them, but we didn't expect to dine out in bistros, brasseries, and cafes.

Of course, we weren't exactly there as tourists, and starting out talking about dining options is known in journalistic circles as "burying the lede." So we'll leave cuisine aside for the moment and get to the heart of the matter.

MD Anderson turned out to be everything everyone said it would. A massive complex packed with patients, doctors, and technicians, Anderson is proof that cancer is big, big business. This is not surprising because, despite all the amazing research being done, and breakthroughs announced or on the horizon, cancer remains a growth industry. We have never been thrilled with the idea of chasing a fad, but still, there was something exciting about being part of an enterprise such as MD Anderson.

We arrived in Houston late Tuesday night thanks to a

three-hour delay in Dallas-Fort Worth. American Airlines was having a really bad hair day, canceling or rescheduling flights and moving them from one gate to another. At the gate next to ours the attendant announced that the flight had been relocated from Gate 27 to Gate 49. All the passengers moved disgruntledly down the hall, including three soldiers dressed in their desert camo. Twenty minutes later they came back.

I asked the soldiers if they really had marched twenty-some gates away only to be sent back to their original gate. Yes, they had. So I told them I hadn't realized the US Army had taken over American Airlines. Lucky for me, they found this remark as amusing as I had expected them to.

But, back to the update. We got to our hotel around 9:30. The restaurant was closed. The last shuttle to Rice Village was about to depart. We caught it, and discovered just about everything there shuts down at 9:00. Luckily there was a Tapas bar open, so we did get to eat.

Next morning we presented ourselves at check-in, where Mary got to fill out reams of reports. Then a brief meeting with Dr. D. before being shunted off for tests. We were done by 4:00 pm Wednesday, with our next appointment not scheduled until Monday afternoon. Which gave us time to explore.

When the time came, we met with Dr. D. again. He reviewed Mary's CT Scan and blood work, which showed her tumors are getting larger and her CEA count continues to rise. No surprises there. After all, that's why we're here. Then came the part where he discussed options. The good news, the main news, is that there are options.

One is to take Regorafenib, or Stivarga, which is an oral treatment. The FDA approved it for treatment of colorectal cancer in 2012. Among its side effects are nausea, fatigue, and hand-foot syndrome. These are similar to what Mary experienced while taking Xeloda last summer. The initial dose made it almost impossible for her to walk, because, she said, it felt like her feet were one giant blister. The lower dose was more tolerable, but it didn't work. Needless to say, she wasn't excited about option number one.

Next on the list: TAS-102. Recently completed Phase III clinical trials show TAS-102 to be effective in extending life, with one-year-survival fifty percent higher for those taking the drug over those receiving a placebo. That the survival rate was only twenty-seven percent gives one pause, but then again, Mary's all about beating the odds.

TAS-102, or Tipiracil Hydrochloride, is a combination of two agents, Trifluridine and Tipiracil Hydrochloride. It is taken orally, once a day for three weeks, then one week off. The drug was first synthesized over fifty years ago, in the form of Trifluridine, but early tests were disappointing. Although the drug was effective in reducing tumors, it had a very short half-life, requiring patients to take a pill every three hours, and it stopped working shortly after the medication ended.

Years later, researchers discovered combining Trifluridine with Tipiracil Hydrochloride served to extend and enhance the drug's effectiveness, which resulted in the FDA putting the drug on a fast track to approval. The target date is in December of this year. In the interim certain cancer centers have been allowed to conduct supplemental clinical trials.

MD Anderson isn't one of those centers, but Karmanos Cancer Center, in the Detroit Medical Center, is. And this is where Dr. D. thinks Mary should go. As he said, "We aren't competing with each other. We all want to cure cancer." It certainly will be more convenient to get treatment fifteen minutes away by car rather than six hours away by plane.

Mary has an appointment with Dr. P. on Monday, at which time we should know if she will be part of the trial. I don't know why she wouldn't be, having achieved refractory status—that's a new term I've learned, it means her cancer isn't responding to any known treatment.

Option three is to look into other clinical trials. Again, Dr. D. recommended Karmanos or University of Michigan, so we'll consider that. The final option, which would have to take place at MD Anderson, is immunotherapy. Dr. D. is going to test on Mary's cancer cells for microsatellite instability, or MSI, which is, of course, a form of genetic hypermutability which results from impaired DNA mismatch repair, or MMR.

The good news is that immunotherapy has a success rate of forty to seventy percent for those with MSI. The bad news is only three to five percent of patients test positive. But, as our old friend Tom Shumaker used to say, Mary isn't interested in those percentages. The only ones that really matter are zero and one hundred percent.

We went like so many others, down to Houston like pilgrims flocking to Lourdes, seeking, if not a cure, at least a way forward. I met a fellow in the hotel bar whose wife is in a clinical trial for breast cancer. He said we were seeking a Silver Bullet. And that's exactly right. And we found our Silver Bullet. Now we can see whether it can hit the heart of this ghoulish cancer, and whether it can strike it dead.

During our time off in Houston, we went shopping, ate French food, spent part of three days at the Houston Museum of Fine Arts. It was interesting to note the similarities between the MFAH and the DIA (Detroit Institute of Art), in terms of the breadth and depth of their collections. It makes sense though, as the impetus for the surge of wealth in Detroit, the auto industry, coincided with the profits of the oilmen who fueled those cars.

We drove to Galveston one afternoon, and went to Needless, where, coincidentally, my sister, Rebecca lived for a few years, to see one of Mary's oldest childhood friends. We had a good old Texas barbecue and enjoyed their down-home hospitality. We had Sunday brunch with Erin, my niece, and only missed Rebecca because she and her husband are traveling in Costa Rica.

I mention all this only to illustrate what Mary said about how much fun it is to travel together. No matter why we find ourselves wherever we are, we both want to get out and explore. Walk or drive around, look at houses and neighborhoods, hit a few gardens and a museum or two, and get a feel for this new city. Oh, and eat.

So we did that, and we learned a lot, and we enjoyed ourselves, and now we are home, ready to begin the next stage of our journey. It's good to know we won't be taking it alone, surrounded as we are with supportive family and friends. Your words of encouragement, your gifts of time and interest, are the dividends Mary has earned for being a good person and a good friend over the course of her life.

Now we're getting ready to fire that Silver Bullet, and hoping the course of her life extends outward as far as the eye can see.

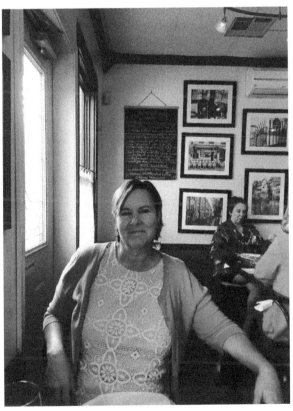

Enjoying dinner at one of Houston's surprising French restaurants.

September 15, 2015
Choices, Choices, Choices

Actually, just two choices, but that's two better than none. After returning from Houston, we met with Dr. P. at Karmanos Cancer Center, in the Detroit Medical Center. We were there to determine whether Mary qualified for adjuvant testing of TAS-102. The initial indications were positive, so we began the process of assembling the myriad of test results and procedures Mary has undergone over the past five years.

One of the most important players was her oncologist, who needed to provide documentation that each of Mary's chemotherapy regimens had eventually failed to work, thereby qualifying her for refractory status, a necessary precursor for taking TAS-102. He sent a terse paragraph in response. Dr. P.'s team required more, so I took on the task of reading through more than five years' of insurance claims (a stack five inches high), to delineate the start and end dates of each treatment and the course of drugs administered during them.

In theory, all those records should have been on a computer, and it would have been the work of a few moments to press the right key and transmit everything to the appropriate office. But no one could be bothered to do that. Apparently, they were so busy resubmitting every one of the last two years' worth of claims to the insurance company that they didn't have time to do the basic research necessary to qualify Mary for a treatment which just might save her life.

It is discouraging, though perhaps not surprising to learn that, though they may at first present themselves as hearty and upbeat, encouraging and seemingly committed to their patient's well-being, or at least survival, at the end of the day medicine is a business, and when doctors can no longer see their patient as a revenue source, then, sometimes they can no longer see their patient.

Or maybe they just grow calloused. Having lost so many patients over the years, maybe they just learn one day that there is a point beyond which they cannot not expend their emotions; there is a point where they have to let go, where they have to stop caring, because caring no longer works.

Maybe that's the case, but they could still could have lifted a finger to help.

At any rate, once the results were compiled and assembled, Mary was told she was likely in. Just one more interview, which took place yesterday, when a nurse came in to ask Mary about herself, and how she was doing. One of the PA's popped in from time to time, "just to listen."

When question time ended, one looked at the other and said, "She's a one?" The other agreed. Mary asked what that meant, and they said it was her ECOG score. They thought one was acceptable, though 0 was preferable. The ECOG score, developed by the Eastern Cooperative Oncology Group, is a scale ranging from zero to five, with zero meaning normal, no complaints, and five standing for dead. A score of one means Mary is "Symptomatic, but completely ambulatory. (Restricted in physically strenuous activity but ambulatory and able to carry out work of a light or sedentary nature. For example, light housework or office work)."

It's rather chilling to see a chart developed to so

clinically gauge a patient's status. But the important thing is, Mary left Karmanos yesterday with a package of pills which she will take, four at a time, morning and evening, for five days. After two days off, she will repeat the dosage. Then, after 16 days off, she will return to Karmanos, have more tests, and get a second dose. This will continue for as long as it is viewed effective.

We're planning for this to go on for quite awhile, as we won't start building our tasting room until next spring, and before that, Mary is taking Emily and Nora to Ireland for a cooking class. (I know, I know, going to Ireland to learn how to cook? I mean, isn't this the place where a plate of French fries and a six-pack of Guinness comprises a seven-course dinner?)

During the run up to the Clinical Trial, Dr. D. called from MD Anderson to say Mary had qualified for a Phase I Clinical Trial. He agreed that she would be better served by beginning the TAS-102 treatment. It was refreshing to have someone view Mary's disease as the focus of treatment, rather than as a revenue stream. Not that Anderson gives their treatment away. They aren't cheap. In fact, they seem to feel they can charge a premium. It will be interesting to see how much our insurance company respects their front-running status.

The bottom line, though, is Mary will be receiving treatment at Karmanos for the time being. Incidentally, yesterday we also got the results of the microsatellite instability test, which, as you may recall, is a form of genetic hypermutability which results from impaired DNA mismatch repair, or MMR. Unfortunately, Mary tested negative, which means she doesn't qualify for this particular form of immunotherapy treatment. Which is a shame, because they are seeing success rates of forty to seventy percent, as opposed to the twenty-seven percent one-year survival rate for TAS-102.

But those are just numbers, and they don't really count. You're either here, or you're not, and nothing else matters. Mary's here, and the quality of her life is good (except for the nagging cough), and we share laughs and sunsets, and two great kids, and scores of wonderful friends. We're still making plans, and that's the important thing.

December 8, 2015
A Day in the Life

Yesterday we drove through thick fog in rush hour traffic to reach Karmanos by 9:00. We had a long day scheduled, maybe four or five hours, we thought, with labs, a CT Scan, and then doctors' appointments. The blood-drawing went off without a hitch, and we left the lab accompanied by a blue-shirted navigator who would guide us through the warrens of the complex to a place called The Rock, where Mary would get her scan.

Only when we got there, the receptionist couldn't find a record of Mary's existence. Her attitude suggested this was somehow Mary's fault. She asked for paperwork and Mary handed over what she had. A few minutes of tapping away at the computer and she said, "Okay, there you are. Just go down this hall, they'll take care of you." She added, looking at me, "You can go too, there's chairs down there."

There were, too, about four of them, each of which had a wheelchair in front of it, on which the wheelchair occupant's companion, looking like he or she should be in one too, was seated. So I wandered back down the hall. No sooner was I settled in than another navigator appeared to tell me my wife was waiting at the end of the hall.

She informed me that this particular CT Scanner wasn't set up to scan clinical trial patients, so we headed back, feeling like rats caught in a maze. Our navigators guided us, and soon we were back on terra firma. We entered a new waiting room where the receptionist seemed much more interested in doing her job. We sat next to Mr. Johnson, who would turn out to be our companion for much of the day. He looked remarkably like Morgan Freeman, and viewed life with a healthy dose of whimsy.

They called his name, I said, "Good luck," and two more patients entered the waiting room. One of them, a young girl in some pain, said she wanted some water. Her mother scowled and growled and finally complied. Then Mr. Johnson came back and said the machine was broken.

We sat there for a couple of hours, while the room steadily filled, while Mr. Johnson's name got called again, and I wished him luck again, and then he returned again because the machine was still broken. We called Angel, Mary's primary nurse, to find out what we should do. She told us to come to the clinic; they'd do her exam and order the next course of medicine, though she couldn't start taking them until after the doctor had reviewed the scan.

We headed to the clinic lobby and waited for them to call Mary's name. Over five-and-a-half years of sitting in chemotherapy labs and cancer clinics, waiting rooms, and lobbies, you get used to seeing things which ordinarily might give you pause. You learn to accept grotesqueries with equanimity.

For some reason on this day, nature pulled out all her stops. Every piece of freak show imagery imaginable was on display. There was the girl in the wheelchair with the face of a woman and the body of a little girl, whose mother rocked her and cooed, and whispered to her. There was the woman in the hijab who stared so boldly and so blatantly at the girl with the face of a woman and the body of a little girl, whose face bore an expression which was in itself a hate crime.

There were the morbidly obese, the painfully bent, the gnarled and twisted, and those of indeterminate sex; they were there en masse, as if depravity had announced a casting call. There was nowhere to avert your eyes, and you felt guilty just for being alive. It was that kind of day. We finally received our summons and went behind the magic wall to visit Mary's nurses and doctors. They reiterated Angel's message that Mary could take the next course with her, but she couldn't start until they saw the results of the CT Scan. Her doctor said she ordinarily didn't like to discuss things like scans over the phone, but she was confident that the results would be good, so if Mary didn't mind, that's what she would do.

Then it was 2:00, and time to return to radiology. Now, Mary had drunk the contrast liquid at 10:00, and hadn't had a bite to eat since 8:00. She couldn't eat now because it might interfere with the scan. When we returned to the waiting room, Mr. Johnson was still there, and greeted us with a rueful smile. But then the preternaturally cheerful nurse popped up to announced that the scanner was finally fixed.

She summoned Mr. Johnson. I told him I wasn't going to wish him good luck this time. He chuckled. And left. And came back ten minutes later as the receptionist got on the phone with Harper Hospital to report our scanner was having "glitches," so could she send some patients over there?

More navigators appeared, pushing wheelchairs for those who needed them. We set off, like refugees from the cancer wars, as we made our way through a warren of subterranean tunnels which connected the entire medical center. When we arrived at Harper's radiology lab, the receptionist acted as if he'd had no warning we were on the way.

One of the patients already waiting there, his skin as black as freshly-laid asphalt, his manner and diction equally evocative of the street, leapt to his feet and asked if we were going to go before him. The receptionist just glared at him, and he replied, "I jes ast one question. Thass all. Damn doctor tryin' to take money from my insurance, sheeit."

Moments later they called his name, and he sprinted for the door, determined not to lose his place in line. While he was gone the rest of the patients got punctured and poked and ready for their own scans. They called Mary's name, so she was gone when the complainer came out. He announced he was gone, "Like a rolling stone," he said. "Like Papa was a rolling stone," he clarified.

"Wherever he laid his hat was his home," I observed.

He turned to me. "You know dat? The Temptations?"

He started to sing. I joined him. We got to "When he died," and I finished with a flourish, "All he left us was alo-o-o-o-o-one." He said, "Oh yeah, you a Detroit boy. Oh yeah."

I glanced over at Mr. Johnson. His bemused expression made him look even more like Morgan Freeman.

Then Mary came out, we said our goodbyes and nine hours after we arrived, we headed back out into the fog and rush hour traffic. We got home around 5:30, and I reheated some spaghetti.

And that's where this one was going to end; only while I was working on it, Mary got a call from the doctor who told her not to take the pills. The scan showed that they aren't working. She says Mary's still in good shape, and she's confident there will be a trial she can take part in. She's got an appointment for next Monday.

We're moving ahead with our Christmas plans. Parties and dinners, and the kids coming down from Traverse City. The house is decorated, and everything looks great, except for the lack of snow. We'll keep moving ahead and defying the future. I'll let you know what next Monday brings.

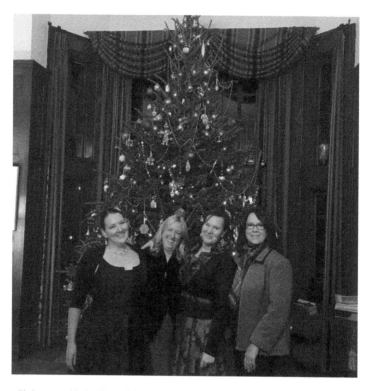

Christmas with family and friends. Emily, Margaret Loomis, Mary, Mary Beth Geltz.

December 22, 2015
Still Laughing

I had a blemish on my face last week, which was threatening to come to a head. Suffice it to say, it wasn't pretty. Since we were getting ready to return to Karmanos Cancer Center, to see what options they might have for Mary, I thought maybe I should put a bandage on my face. Or not, I mused. Maybe they would see it and inform me I had megalomaniacalsarcomaticmelanoma or something, to which Mary replied, "Oh no you don't. You're not dying before me."

And I said, "More than five-and-a-half years in, and we're still joking about cancer."

Which is probably one reason Mary's still here five-and-a-half years later. I can't say she doesn't take it seriously, because it's hard not to, but she refuses to let it wear her down. We could all learn from her. I could learn from her. I wish I had last Tuesday when I broke down and cried on her shoulder. I apologized. She said it was okay. But it wasn't.

I tried to explain it to my friend Dave, whom I see once a year during the holidays, and he gives me an update on his cancer, and I give him one on Mary's, when he told me it was okay, saying, "I probably cry once every three days."

"It's okay for you to cry," I said. "You have cancer. But it's not okay for me to cry, because that means I've given up, and the only job I have is to believe."

Anyway, we went back to Karmanos, and things worked more smoothly. Dr. P. was back, though still fighting a cold. He told us, after reviewing the CT Scan, that he wanted Mary to stay on the medication. Even though a couple of the tumors had grown, including the one in her lung which encroaches on her air passage and causes her to cough, most of the others stayed the same size.

He explained that with this drug they don't really look for shrinkage, and, frankly, there just aren't any good alternatives out there. So Mary's back on the best option available. It may not be working perfectly, but it's doing its primary job, which is keeping her alive.

We had our Christmas party last Saturday. Emily's friend Claire, and our friend Katharine came over to help Mary and Emily with the preparations. It was good they were both there, because Mary took a couple of breaks, which she's never ever done before. But she stayed on her feet until we said goodbye to the last of the guests (except for those who didn't leave for hours) sometime after midnight.

As I clarified to the doctor when he asked Mary if she had energy, and she said, no, not really, her energy is good. It just doesn't last very long. But this is our new normal. Short-term plans include Christmas with the kids, a trip for Mary to Arizona in February, and then down to Florida with friends. March is cooking in Ireland with Emily and Nora, and then, in April, a friend's daughter's destination wedding in sunny Mexico.

Those are the plans. I expect us to keep them.

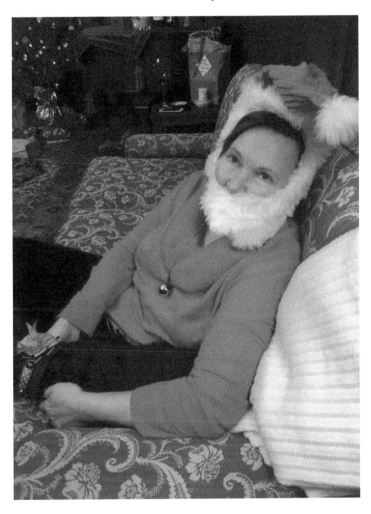

January 15, 2016
That Boat Has Already Sailed

On January 28, Mary will undergo a surgical procedure called Endobronchial Argon Plasma Coagulation, which involves inserting a tube called a bronchoscope into her lung, expelling some argon gas which is then zapped with a high-voltage electric current. If all goes well, this should result in the breakup of a tumor in her right lung which is currently encroaching on her air passage, causing a really painful sounding cough, and interfering with her ability to breathe.

We got the ball rolling this week when we met with Dr. S., the Karmanos Cancer Center lung specialist, who after examination recommended a course of radiation. Naturally, Mary was concerned about when this could start and how long it would last, pointing out that we had plans to go to Arizona and Florida next month.

I suggested perhaps fixing her lungs might have a higher priority. The attending health care specialists seemed to agree with me. Anyway, after exploring our options, it looked like the course would be finished before the middle of next month, so our travel plans were intact, except for a visit Up North to taste our wine and help make a final determination on the style we wanted to see in the bottle, which we would have to cancel.

Unfortunately, the next day, the radiation specialist, Dr. P., told us he couldn't provide radiation, because of serious and potentially fatal side effects arising from her previous courses of Avastin. So it was back to the drawing board, with a new doctor, and a new procedure.

It was during her meeting with Dr. S. that Mary mentioned she sometimes coughed up blood. That was one of the reasons the doctors and nurses were so intent on finding a treatment for her. It was also the first time I had heard about it.

Mary said she didn't want to tell me, because she didn't want me to worry. I told her, "That ship sailed a long time ago." And it has. In case you're wondering, it's not a cruise ship, rather a battleship, and it keeps circling the harbor, firing salvos of dread and despair at the hapless defendants.

Having been downtown most of this past week, we've taken advantage of it by finally starting to hit some of Detroit's myriad new restaurants for lunch. It's something new, this knowing there are some restaurants we'll never get to. It's been a long, long time since Detroit has had this sort of problem.

So, this is how we live now, making the best of the situation, trying to find opportunities in the challenges; making plans, sometimes changing them, sometimes canceling. Mary suggested maybe we could fly from Arizona, where we would be staying with Wendy and Tom, straight to Florida, to meet Mark and Molly and Bryan and Rachel in three days' time. I suggested we could rent a car, maybe drive to Miami, see my Uncle Peter, or go to Key West, which I've never seen.

Mary listened to my planning, not really commenting, as she does sometimes. So I asked her if she had a problem with it. After all, it was her idea. She said she wasn't sure. Maybe she wouldn't feel well enough to go. I told her we should just make our plans. We can cancel them if we have to. Because, that's what you do.

Anyway, that's the plan. Surgery on the 28th. It's supposed to be pretty basic, an outpatient procedure. But I doubt we'll be checking out one of the new restaurants that day.

I'll keep you posted. Don't be afraid to drop by or call.

January 28, 2016
My, That Was Fun

Today was basically a good news/bad news sort of day. The good news? Mary went under, underwent the procedure, and came back to us. The bad news? She has to do it again, at least one more time.

You've heard the saying, that was fun, let's do it again. That's pretty much what Dr. J. told me this afternoon after Mary's procedure. He said it was successful, with no complications or other problems. He did say the tumor was larger than he expected, and had almost completely closed one airway. It was too large to handle in one procedure, so he would like to do it again, maybe next Thursday, if there is an OR opening.

He stressed that he wouldn't suggest this if he didn't think it would do some good. Which means, basically, he is optimistic. It's hard to tell sometimes with Dr. J. He doesn't give a lot away. Sort of like Dr. House, I suppose, without the cane. But at least he thought things over before he started cutting. (I know if I were ever in the emergency room with some non-defined malady and I saw Dr. House enter the room, I would flee, because he would immediately diagnose some rare disease, amputate my leg, remove my spleen, accidentally blind me, and then decide it was "just a cold." But I don't think he's on the air any more, so we're probably safe).

Anyway, we'll do this a couple more times, and if all is successful, Mary won't be coughing as much, and the quality of her life will greatly improve.

As we got Mary prepared for surgery, as a steady stream of nurses, doctors, interns, and trainees passed through the room, asking her the same questions, and making the same notes on the same sheets of paper, it struck me again what amazing people nurses are. For the last almost six years we have been meeting all kinds of nurses as Mary has undergone a vast array of procedures and processes, and all of them, male or female, have been so kind, so considerate, so ready and willing to put her at ease (and to tell me to just shut up). They are a rare breed. Nursing is a gift, and we are lucky to be beneficiaries.

While Mary was in surgery, I got to meet Nanci Burrows, the Karmanos Cancer Center Director of Customer Service, who had received a copy of my horrible, awful, no good day at Karmanos update. She had called, apologized, and promised to get to the bottom of things. I stressed at the time that I hadn't written it to complain, rather just to share a day-in-the-life-of experience, and that what made the day so bad was not the experience itself, but the bad news at the end of it.

I also told her I would be satisfied if Karmanos would give a copy of my novel to each new patient. She asked me about it, and I gave her a brief description. Then she asked if I thought it would help the patients. I replied, "I don't know. I just want to sell a lot of copies."

Well, she came to visit me in the waiting lounge today, and bought a copy of *Rebound*. Which I thought was very nice. No word on whether Karmanos will be buying several thousand copies, but don't hold your breath.

I'll let you know what next week will bring, but in the meantime, thanks so much for your thoughts, prayers, hopes, and words of encouragement. They mean so much and they last so long.

February 5, 2016
Thank You, We'll Be Here All Week

Mary underwent her second Endobronchial Argon Plasma Coagulation. (Incidentally, I thought I was going to have to publicly correct myself, because everybody kept referring to it as a laser procedure, while my understanding was they didn't use laser any more—however, yesterday just before they wheeled Mary into the Operating Room, Dr. J. responded impatiently to someone who used the term laser, saying, "It's not laser. I wish people would quit saying it is." Ah, vindication. Never gets old).

While we were waiting in the pre-op room for the team to get settled, Mary's nurse came in to explain why she had to take more blood. For some reason, the pre-admission blood tests taken at Karmanos are good for a month, but post-admission blood taken at Harper expires in three days. Mary and I glanced at each other. The nurse said, "What?"

And Mary, right on cue, said, "Never say 'expire' to a patient in the Operating Room."

That took me back to the wit she flashed at her first surgery, when friends said, "We'd better go. I think they want to close these curtains," and she said, "Never say curtains in the operating room," and, laughing, one of them said, "Okay, we'll see you on the other side," and she said, "Never say on the other side..."

A rare talent, this OR Standup, especially since she had to do the Standup lying down.

So, we had that going for us. And a nurse willing to share a laugh with us. An hour or so later, the doctor came out to tell me the procedure was a success, he had opened two air passages, and there was no need to do anything else at this time. He has no need to see Mary, but she should feel free to call him with any questions.

It took about an hour longer this week for Mary to recover enough to go home, but she bounced back in the evening and had a very good appetite. Today we went back to Karmanos where she had an appointment with an Ear, Nose, and Throat specialist who prescribed some pills and thought even though her cough probably was caused by her lung tumors, there was enough congestion in her head and throat that it likely exacerbated the problem.

Between the new medication, and her rapid recovery today, we're fairly optimistic that her cough will be, if not defeated, certainly beaten well back. Which will be a very good outcome indeed. In fact, except for that whole incurable cancer thing, she's in really good shape.

We're looking forward to finishing the month with trips to Arizona and Florida, and in just four weeks, celebrating her sixth anniversary. Never thought we'd get there, and haven't felt this positive about pushing the finish line further down the road for quite some time.

March 10, 2016
Thank You, God

We had the opportunity to spend a long weekend with our friends down in Florida, so naturally, we took it. A beautiful home, on Sanibel Island, with access to the beach through a wild stretch of seaside vegetation. Mary told me one day, while she was walking through this miniature jungle, she stopped and said a prayer.

"I said 'Thank you, God, for letting me come here.' For this weekend, our friends, just for everything."

"Everything, except the cancer," I said.

"No, I even thanked Him for the cancer. It has made me appreciate life so much."

I guess it does do that; it helps you focus. And we have been the recipients of that distinctive outlook for six years now. Or, to put it in perspective, Mary has now survived a full five years longer than the one year her original Dr. Doom gave her. So, yes, let's be grateful. And let's continue to accept those invitations, no matter how distant, no matter how far away.

We were looking at a destination wedding in Cancun, at

the end of April. Mary said she wasn't sure. It was too far in the future to plan with confidence. So I said we'd buy trip insurance. And we did, and we're going.

We had a setback of sorts, a couple weeks ago, in the treatment realm, when, after Mary's successful bronchoscopies, Dr. P. said he didn't think she should go back on Lonsurf, because it wasn't fully working. This was the opposite of what he'd said before the procedures, but I'm getting used to this by now. Anyway, he suggested something called Stivarga, which is similar to Xeloda, the drug which didn't really work for Mary but gave her serious foot and hand pain.

First, he said, he wanted to do a CT Scan. This was on a Monday in mid-February. Mary was very much hoping to leave that Thursday for Tucson. Luckily, we managed to snag a spot on Wednesday, so she could have her scan and beat it, too.

The next Monday we were back at Karmanos, at 2:15. At 3:15 we were still waiting. At 3:30 we were dumped in a room where we were informed Dr. P. wouldn't be seeing Mary, but his assistant would be. At 4:15 a Nurse Practitioner came in, introduced herself and proceeded to ask all the questions a health care provider asks during an introductory visit.

I started to get the sense that the CT Scan wasn't very positive, and that Dr. P. was basically punting on Mary. That sense grew when the nurse said Dr. P. had left us with two options at the last visit, and she was wondering which one we'd chosen.

This was a tad confusing as neither Mary nor I remembered receiving that assignment. He did suggest Stivarga, I said.

"Stivarga?" she said, sounding perplexed. That wasn't one of the options.

"Well, maybe you can find someone who is familiar with Mary's case," I suggested.

She did, eventually, manage to locate Dr. P., who made an appearance around 5:00, and told Mary he didn't think

Stivarga was a very good idea, that it probably wouldn't work, and what she needed to do was try to get into a Phase 1 Clinical Trial.

We had that appointment last week, where we met the staff and learned the ins and outs, of Clinical Trials. We also learned that because of the length and progression of Mary's disease, she doesn't qualify for second or third phases, only for the preliminary trials. Dr. W. was very informative, very professional, and promised their Clinical Trial committee would review Mary's status, and have an answer for us by this week.

So we went back this past Tuesday to learn that there isn't anything suitable right now. There is a promising immunotherapy trial which should be starting in two months or so, and Mary is on a wait list for that one. Not the best of developments, but the good news is Mary still feels pretty good, her cough, while still harsh and present, has diminished some since her procedures. It doesn't impose itself on her as much, and as a result, her spirits are far, far better than they were a month ago. As she says, "I feel like it's given me months."

Next week we'll go back to see Dr. P., or whichever surrogate he deems appropriate, and find out if, as Dr. W. suggested, Mary starts taking Stivarga. In the meantime, it might be time for another call to MD Anderson, to see if they have any clinical trials for us to consider.

But here's a thought to leave you with in closing. If Mary can thank God for her cancer, surely there are many more things you can be thankful for, as well.

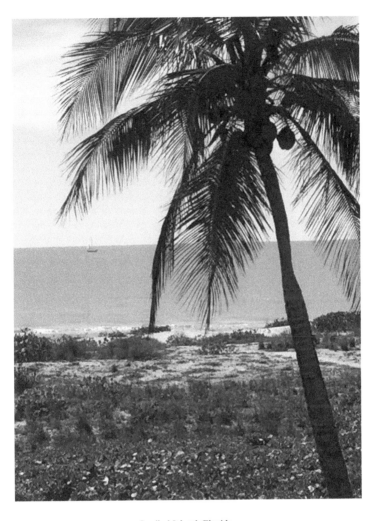

Sanibel Island, Florida

April 15, 2016
Don't Put It Off

So these are the days of long constraint, of late night wakening and sudden sorrows. These are the days when, if someone asks you how you're doing, and it seems everybody does, you sigh and say "All right." These are the days when you gather strength from a gesture, a pat on the back, a note in the mail, a pot of white chicken chili that magically appears in the fridge while you were at a movie (with tears clouding your eyes because you looked at the laughable old couple in the silly rom-com, and thought how unfair that you would not be growing old together like that).

We went to see Dr. D. at Karmanos Cancer Center. He is a supportive care doctor, the specialist who helps you when nobody else can. The one who brings in hospice, at the end. Mary asked, "Realistically, how long have I got." He said, "We should think in months, not years." He also said if we had any plans, we shouldn't put them off.

That's hard to take, but it is something we always knew was there. High fives and trash-talking cancer was fun, and laughing in cancer's face was cathartic, but we also knew cancer has a way of biding its time. It didn't need to claim its pound of flesh all at once. It was content to lie in wait, confident at some point we would lay down our guard, and then it would pounce.

Mary has a lost a lot of weight, and looks really good, right now. But satisfying as it might be to lose weight without trying, there is something disconcerting about it, too. It means yes, something is very wrong.

She has started a new drug called Stivarga. The doctor said it's not meant to cure her cancer, at best it will retard the tumors' growth. It comes with a long list of side effects, far more than Lonsurf, that clinical trial she was on, the placeholder drug that's supposed to take Stivarga's place. The one that didn't work for her. So far, the side effects have been mild, and Mary will tell you she believes it is working. She can feel it, she says. Which is nice to hear.

A woman from the pharmaceutical company told me Blue Cross Blue Shield said there would be a $600 copay for the drug. I asked how that could be since we had already reached the maximum out of pocket expense. She told me she had asked the same question, and was told, "I don't know, maybe it's a penalty or something."

So I called Blue Cross Blue Shield and quoted that remark. I said, "I don't know, maybe it's me, but I think having cancer is penalty enough. You don't have to go around adding more."

I kept asking how there could be a copay when we had already reached our maximum out-of-pocket expense. She kept trying to come up with something that sounded good. I finally said, "Maybe it's a language thing. I'm dealing with English, in which maximum means the most you have to pay. But maybe in insurance language maximum means the very least you can expect to pay. Is that what it is? A language problem?"

She said she'd get back to me. I said, "Yeah, right," because that's what they all say to get me off the phone. She actually seemed offended, repeating, "I said I will call you back." She sounded even more offended two hours later when I told her how surprised I was that she actually had called back. It was as if I had impugned her integrity. Who knew?

Anyway, she concluded we didn't have to pay a copay, because we had, in fact, met our maximum out-of-pocket expense. It's always nice when you win one, though sometimes it would be nice not to have to fight them.

Last weekend, Mary helped put on a tea for fifty at the Ford House. It was the annual Herb Society tea. A speaker came in from Virginia and stayed at our house for three days. Mary was very busy, though she had more help than she usually does for this kind of event. She was up early and stayed up all day. I kept expecting her to crash. She never did. Sunday afternoon we were supposed to visit friends for a cocktail. I fully expected to call and cancel. But we didn't. I started thinking maybe I was too pessimistic. Maybe she had more in reserve than I thought. The next day she was supposed to go to Partridge Creek to look for resort wear for our trip to Cancun at the end of the month. She was going to leave at 10:00. Then 11:00. Then, she thought, maybe 1:00. Since she was still in her nightgown, I suggested maybe it was okay if she didn't go that day. Maybe it was okay if she did nothing all day.

We went on Wednesday, and walked in and out of a bunch of stores. She didn't buy anything. Today she's going to another mall with a friend to walk around and look at more clothes. I told her it would have been a very disappointing trip if that had happened to me, but she seemed to feel it was a successful day. I think I've actually shopped successfully maybe three times in my life.

So, the trip to Cancun is still on. We received an invitation to another destination wedding, this one at Lake Tahoe, in July. It came with a beautiful note from the bride-to-be, about the inspiration Mary's courage and grace has given her, and how she wants our relationship to be the standard she and her husband aspire to in their own marriage.

It made me cry.

We're thinking about that one. Maybe. It's not far from my folks, so we could go to the wedding and spend a couple days in Lodi. If Mary's up to it. We'll buy trip insurance again, because that's how we do it now. It's tough not knowing whether Mary will be up to it, but like the doctor said, we'll keep making plans.

April 27, 2016
Adios, Cancun

We were supposed to fly to Cancun today, for Jean and Chris' wedding. Instead, we're at home, monitoring Mary's condition, trying to decide whether to go to the hospital, trying to decide if the nurse we saw Monday is right, and these are side effects of Stivarga, or if Mary is right and there's some serious blockage inside her. She was certainly right about running a fever, and the nurse appeared to be more invested in accurate note taking than in the well-being of her patient.

Maybe Mary is just fighting a bug, on top of everything else. After all, the fever seems to have broken last night. This all started last Tuesday, when she woke up in serious pain. Gas pains, she called it. Maybe yes, maybe no. Our friends James and Sophie came in from Montreal on Wednesday, for the Racquets Weekend at the DRC, and there was a whole series of events planned. Mary made most of them, though often not for long, and often not until the last minute, when she decided she was strong enough to attend.

Then, on Sunday, she failed to answer the bell. She didn't feel up to getting out of bed. She was in pain, and nauseous, and didn't want to eat or drink. We thought about the hospital, but didn't know which one we should go to, and no one was returning our calls. Finally, we called Katherine, a friend, and nurse practitioner, who came over and got Mary to drink some liquids, showing me in the process that I shouldn't be so respectful of Mary's wishes. If she needs to eat or drink, she has to.

Now Katherine's style is one of cajoling and couching requests in the form of a challenge. "I bet you can take another three sips of water," and things like that. Me, I went for barking orders. Yesterday morning I scrambled an egg for Mary. She sat with it in front of her for awhile. "Eat your eggs!" I commanded. She looked at me, rolled her eyes, and said, "Did you really think that was going to work?" But she did eat some.

It was great to spend time with James and Sophie. I told Mary, Monday morning while driving to Karmanos for a handful of appointments and what turned into two hours in the infusion center on a saline drip to rehydrate her, how much strength I'd gained from their visit.

Eight hours later, driving away from the center, all that strength was gone. So much so that, after sitting behind a car which failed to move for most of a green light, and then slid indifferently into the left turn lane, oblivious to my screaming "Quit your damn texting!" I pulled up next to him and glared at him until Mary said, "Oh, please don't get into a fight!" Highly unlikely that, since it would have required the guy to look up from his phone, and who wants to do that in the middle of rush hour traffic?

So, here's a tip to keep in mind if you ever find yourself in our situation. If they ask you if you want to watch TV when they usher you into the examination room, you can bet you're going to be there for a long, long time before some CPN comes in and tells you she's up to speed on your case because she sat across the table from one of the other nurses at lunch last Friday.

Which treatment kind of makes me think maybe it isn't

a side effect, and maybe it isn't a bug, but maybe we're starting the homestretch, and this is the way it's going to be from now on, however long now on will be, and it won't be pleasant, and it won't be pretty.

I wouldn't mind being wrong. After all, there are some arguments you just don't want to win. We'll know more in the next few days. If it's a bug or side effects, Mary will start to get better. If it isn't, she won't, and then we shall see what we shall see.

May 16, 2016
Amazing Grace

My last post ended on a down beat. It was written without a lot of enthusiasm, and with less hope. The following week suggested, if anything, I had succumbed to an excess of optimism. That week was, without question, the worst of Mary's life. It seemed we were spending half our time at the Karmanos Acute Care Center, where Mary received infusions of painkillers and saline solution to rehydrate her.

She couldn't, or wouldn't eat, because food made her sick, and it hurt her to swallow, so she wasn't drinking enough fluids. It was on Monday, May 2 that she hit bottom. She was crying out in pain. This is a woman who gave birth to two children without making a sound, and she was crying out in pain. We kept wondering whether to go to an emergency room, and if so, which one.

Eventually, though, morning came, and we drove to the clinic, and they started doing things that made her feel better. Dr. D., the supportive care specialist came in. He prescribed a stronger dose of morphine to manage Mary's general pain, with norco to address more acute pain. He also suggested hospice. He said hospice gets a bad rep, with people assuming they only come in at the very end. That's not true, he observed. They come in when there is nothing left to do, but that doesn't mean it's the end.

So Mary got out of the hospital that Tuesday, and by Wednesday morning two very worried kids and one worried daughter-in-law were burning up the airwaves and texting up a blizzard trying to find out what was going on. This is what happens when you leave someone like me in charge of communications.

After that horrible night on the 2nd, I wasn't sure Mary would survive until Friday, when the kids were planning to come down from Traverse City, for a rugby match and Mother's Day Brunch. So I texted a heads up to them from the hospital. Once Mary had stabilized and it looked like things were going to be okay, I relaxed. Relaxing is good. Completely forgetting to let them know things were better? Not so good.

The weekend was very nice. We collaborated on Mother's Day Brunch, after everyone went to church together. Better than any restaurant in town was my verdict, though the string quartet or soft jazz combo was noticeable by their absence.

Before the weekend, however, we got to work on necessary housekeeping. We met with Pastor Justin to review funeral plans. When discussing possible hymns, neither Mary nor I could come up with the name, "Amazing Grace," which was ironic since it was while singing that hymn, some six years ago, we realized there is no such thing as information management. Everybody will know soon enough that you have cancer. Cancer doesn't just move into your house; cancer becomes the house you live in. We realized that because by the end of the hymn we both had tears streaming down our cheeks, and it was obvious to everyone around us that something was wrong.

That something is more wrong now than ever before, but thanks to this new drug regimen, Mary feels more comfortable. Her appetite is back, though her sense of humor, sadly has not returned. I'm delivering some of my best material and, nothing. She doesn't laugh. She doesn't react at all, except for a brief roll of the eyes and a martyred shrug. Come to think of it, that's how she's always reacted...

Seriously, two weeks ago we were discussing the likelihood of her still being here when my parents came to visit at the end of the month. She thought maybe she would be. "Then our next target is our anniversary, June 12th," I said.

"I don't think I'll make it that far."

Now, however, we're making plans for that day. So we have been granted an amazing grace period. For how long, who knows. But we'll keep taking it until it stops coming. We went Up North last week, to see the lake house, and the vineyard. At first, it was just a distant goal that we could go. Then, when it appeared likely it would work, it assumed in our minds the stature of a poignant tour, a chance to say goodbye. By the time we headed back downstate on Friday, we were already making plans for when we would return.

So there is hope, in the short term. Yesterday we were back at Karmanos for a follow-up visit with Dr. R., the oral doctor, who had prescribed a drug to deal with the sore on her gum. One doctor, a periodontist, had been afraid to touch it, theorizing it might be cancer. Others, dentists, and Dr. R., discounted that likelihood. Yesterday he said he didn't like the way it was growing. It didn't look like an infection, so he was going to take a biopsy.

It really doesn't matter, was basically what he told us, since even if it were cancer, they probably wouldn't do anything to treat it. I asked if he suspected that it was further metastization. He didn't know. It could be an entirely new cancer, but it wouldn't change things. The treatment would involve rather serious surgery, major discomfort, and it wouldn't have any effect on the underlying condition.

We're going back to Karmanos to see Dr. D. on Thursday, with a stop on the way at Elmwood Cemetery to pick out a plot. By then we should know if the biopsy is positive or negative.

But let me leave you on a positive note. When Emily was here before Mother's Day she accompanied us to the funeral home so Mary could pick out her casket and funeral arrangements—okay, maybe it doesn't sound all that positive, but work with me on this one. We looked at different plans, and different price ranges, and then we went into the showroom where we could see the actual coffins. We looked at prayer cards and visitation options, and discussed all the various logistics of the "death care industry."

When we were finally done, with everything in place, Mary said, "Yay," which is how she always characterizes a successful shopping outing. And that's the spirit we're going to keep going as long as we possibly can.

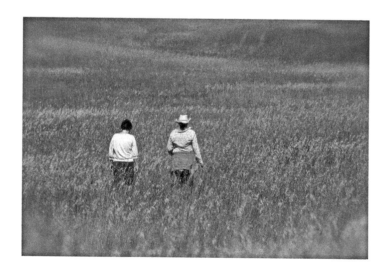

May 25, 2016
A Little of This, A Little of That

There have been good days and bad days. Good days, when friends make a point of calling, then dropping by, or sending flowers, or inviting themselves over for dinner, and bringing dinner with them. And bad days, when Mary can't get out of bed, and feels guilty for "being so lazy." "I feel like I'm sleeping my whole life away," she complained the other day.

That's one way of looking at it, I thought. Another is you're sleeping away so you can enjoy the life you have left.

Last Thursday was a not so good day because Dr. D. shared the biopsy report with us. This is the one from the sore in Mary's mouth, the one that half the experts thought might be, and the other half were adamant it wasn't cancer. Well, it was. Not much they can do about it. Maybe radiation for palliative purposes.

Then somebody in the field told me hospice often doesn't like it if the patient undergoes radiation. I said it wasn't curative treatment. He said it didn't matter. It wasn't a procedural issue as much as a financial one. Apparently, hospice is paid for their services, and treatments like radiation come out of their share. Well, maybe we won't go that route, then. After all, it has been Mary's goal ever since she got diagnosed with cancer to make sure as many people could get as wealthy as possible.

Yesterday was a good day. Mary went to book club, then in the evening there was a reception at the Services For Older Citizens, or SOC Center, where Mary and her friend Molly had designed a culinary herb garden. One of the members of the Herb Society thought it would be a good idea to present her with a commemorative bench. About fifty people were there, on a perfect evening. Mary was suitably gratified. She made a gracious speech. How much nicer it is to be present at the installation of a commemorative bench than to be remembered with a memorial one.

Also yesterday I received a called from Karmanos regarding a Phase 1 Clinical Trial that has opened up. It involves immunotherapy, the Holy Grail of cancer research. There haven't been a lot of immunotherapy options for colorectal cancer, so this would represent cutting-edge treatment, with a chance for substantial and dramatic improvement.

Mary qualifies genetically. Whether she does physically is open to question. She has an appointment on June 14th with Dr. W., the Clinical Trial doctor, to see if she is in good enough shape to handle the treatment. Of course, we will want to know as much about the process as possible. Even if she qualifies, she may not want to do it. Mary's first reaction when I told her about it was, "They want me to take another drug?" Her experience with Stivarga has put her off drugs, at least for the time being.

In a way, this last-second extension of a sliver of hope reminds me of those old melodramatic serials, which used to play in what were known as movie houses, each episode of which would end with our heroine tied to the railroad tracks, a locomotive charging down the track at her. (I read a book about the history of cinema, that's how I know about this. How old do you think I am?) Anyway, here we are at death's door, and Dudley Do-Right comes racing in to save the day. Or not. Time will tell.

Meanwhile, my parents arrive for a few days' visit tonight, then Mary Lou and Cordelia, two of Mary's old college friends will be here for a few days. I will take advantage of the latter interlude to head Up North for some intensive work with weed whacker, chain saw, mower, and hoe. Mary will join me on the 6th for a few days.

We continue to make plans, because that's what you do. Don't be afraid to visit. Call first, to see if Mary is up to it. Don't be offended if the answer is no. It's nothing personal (in most cases), just not the right day. Thanks for being there to support us. It means more than you will ever know.

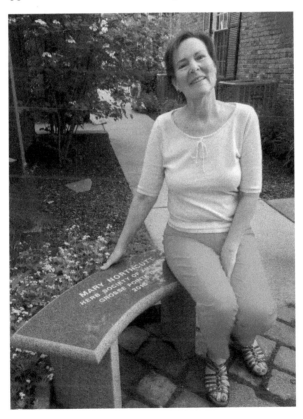

June 16, 2016
Such a Complainer

It has been a busy three weeks since my last update. My parents came in for a five-day visit from California, followed by Mary Lou and Cordelia, two of Mary's friends from college days. I picked them up from the airport and left town the next day to go Up North and put some much-needed work in the vineyard and grounds, leaving them to spend some quality, though sadly also good-bye time together.

Back when I first got to know then like then love Mary, Mary Lou and Cordelia and I didn't exactly get along. It was some years later when we finally understood we had all been jealous of Mary's affections. They didn't want to lose her to "some boy," and I didn't want to share her attention with anyone. It's nice to know we can change and improve as we grow more mature.

When they left, our friend Rachel drove Mary up to Glen Lake, where she stayed for a couple of days. Mary and I remained until our return trip Saturday. We spent one afternoon at the brand spanking new Cowell Family Cancer Center in Traverse City when Mary hit another low hydration wall. A doctor friend in town made some calls which allowed us to get into the infusion center without long delays or another blizzard of paperwork.

Matthew, Nora, and Emily spent the next three nights at Glen Lake, spending valuable one-on-one time with their mother and mother-in-law. It is heartbreaking to realize every interaction has a valedictory air about it these days.

We drove home on Saturday, taking a three-hour detour so Mary could visit Pond Hill Farm, north of Harbor Springs. Driving up the Michigan coast is such a wonderful experience. It is truly beautiful countryside, very settled and tamed in the English manner, with blocks of wildness interspersed. People with vision have done their part to ensure that much of what remains will continue to do so as the landscape is dotted with signs declaring this stand of trees, that meadow, and the marshland next to it are designated nature preserves.

We had a long drive home, and the following day, our anniversary, we spent alone, at home. I recalled, vaguely as in the distant past, our night on the town for Valentine's Day, staying at the aLoft Hotel on Grand Circus Park, and having dinner at Joe Muers. Was it really just four months ago? We watched a James Bond marathon. It's what you do for your 34th. Go ahead, check the traditional anniversary gift chart. 25th is silver, 30th is pearl, and 34th is vodka, shaken, not stirred.

On Monday, Mary had an appointment with Dr. R. to review the Cat Scan of her jaw and discuss options. It was set for 8:45. Unfortunately, we had to cancel. Mary couldn't answer the bell. In fact, she didn't get up until around 4:00 pm. She was up much of the night coughing and taking various medications while I lay in bed wondering if she would make it through the week, and if she had bought my Father's Day gift early.

When I got up the next day, I found an email from my sister informing me that my father was in the hospital with a series of bacteriological infections. Sometimes you just laugh, because that's all they've left you.

That afternoon we met with Dr. W. to discuss the immunotherapy trial. At first, she was all gung-ho about getting Mary started, well, maybe after a course of radiation to reduce the tumor in her mouth. Okay, maybe, upon consideration, we should think this through. Basically, what it comes down to, is even though Mary qualifies genetically, she really isn't strong enough to survive the treatment.

That was one of the reasons we kept the appointment, out of curiosity as to what it would entail. And Dr. W. told us. It would take about three months of unpleasantness before any positive results would show, if any positive results would show. She would get worse before she got better, and we reluctantly agreed Mary couldn't afford to get much worse. But we made a follow-up appointment in a month, and if Mary rallies and is so inclined, she can still get into the trial. Had a bit of the wink-wink, nudge-nudge to it, that last bit.

Today we saw Dr. D., the supportive care physician. He is a unique figure, so somber; it's as if he is absorbing the weight of his patient's pain. Mary asked him if he was able to turn it off when he went home. He said he tried to. We discussed Mary's condition, worsening, and her options, not so many, and not so rosy. He used the term tipping point in reference to her chances of getting strong enough to enter the trial.

We talked about an interview with hospice. We talked about the tumor in her mouth. We looked at the strange lump on her shin. I would point to places on her body and remind her to mention what was going on there. It was around then that Mary apologized, "I'm sorry to be such a complainer," she said.

I remember once hearing a violinist draw high notes of such exquisite clarity from the strings that my eyes watered, without reference to my emotional state. I'm pretty sure it was the same case at that instance, something about the sound of her voice at the perfect pitch, that's what made my eyes well up. I'm sure of it.

So, we are well into those days of days. It is a matter of days, or weeks, or months. We don't know. It's the knowing but not knowing which is the hardest part. On her good days, we still make plans. On her bad days, she wonders why she bothers.

Somebody told me he thought in some ways it must be harder on me than on her. I thought, "No, it's not even close."

June 28, 2016
Don't Be Sad

"Don't be sad." That's what Mary told Dr. D. when he dropped in for a visit before she got discharged from the hospital yesterday. His demeanor is one of empathetic sadness. It is as if he is absorbing all his patient's pain and sorrow.

"Don't be sad," she told him yesterday. "I've had a wonderful six years."

Last Thursday, we went to Karmanos for a consultation with Dr. P., the radiation oncologist. The plan was to do a course of radiation on her jaw before we brought in hospice, but the consultation turned into a more wide-ranging examination, and when he heard about her fall the week before, coupled with the weakness in her legs, the doctor ordered an emergency MRI.

Then followed a few hours of being shunted from hallway to hallway, room to room, with some nurses not quite successfully communicating with other nurses. Finally, she disappeared through the doorway to the big magnetic machine, and I went to get a bite to eat.

When I returned she was lying on a bed, rather loopy, and no one really saying much of anything. Finally one of the nurses explained we were waiting for a room to open and someone from transport to take her there. Turns out they were admitting her, but no one could say why.

We got to the room. The nurses were, as nurses usually are, cheerful and helpful, but no one could explain why she'd been admitted. Finally around 9:00, a doctor came in and explained that the cancer had gone to Mary's spine, and there were three small fractures. They were going to start radiation on her jaw the next day, and run CT Scans so they could set up a framework for spinal radiation as well.

Matt and Nora had come down to spend the weekend with Mary and ended up sharing time with her in her room. Actually, Nora subbed for Mary at the Garden Center's Garden Tour. She had been scheduled to work at one of the houses as cashier from 1:00 to 4:00 on Friday. I thought it might be nice if Nora could be there with her, since she wouldn't be able to do it herself. As it turned out, Nora ended up doing it alone.

Saturday another doctor came in and informed me that the cancer was in Mary's brain. I sort of thought it might be, given Mary's intermittent lucidity. She, of course, maintained it was Matthew and I who were having lucidity problems. She was perfectly fine.

Sunday was another story. I went to church. People asked about Mary. I tried to give them an update, but suddenly I found it hard to talk, or breathe, or see, for that matter. It was as if I were seeing everything from underwater. Weird, huh? I saw Bill Wrobel, and he gave me a big hug, and I cried a little, but was unable to say what I wanted to say, which was, that Mary had held it at bay for six years, but now it was in control. Cancer was taking a victory lap. Cancer was having its revenge. A vengeful beast, cancer is.

But when I got to the hospital, Mary was much, much better. So much so that Matt and Nora, who had decided not to return to Traverse City, decided they could, and did, with my blessings. Monday she went for radiation, and then we sat around for hours waiting for the doctor who was coming to fit her with a back brace. He finally showed up around 5:00, and we were out of there around 6:00 pm.

Laura was there to meet us, and Margaret had brought milkshakes by. We watched the Detroit fireworks on tv, reminiscing about the times when we went downtown to see them. A spectacular show, even though television can never do them justice. The picture was on the screen; the sound came through the window ten seconds later.

Then this morning Mary was very tired, and not too connected to reality. Laura and Therese came over, just about the time I completely lost it. After trying for a couple of hours to get Mary dressed to make her radiation appointment, I realized there really wasn't any use in trying to get there. I called. They called back, and we agreed it's time to bring in hospice.

Maybe she'll continue to alternate, good days for bad. Maybe hospice can get her medications right. Maybe we can go on for a little while longer.

July 1, 2016
A Mary-Sized Hole

Someone said, "It's nice the weather cooperated," as we awoke to a gray, rainy day. The house has been filled with friends, family, and well-wishers these past few days, in a sort of rolling pre-wake celebration of Mary and her life and the impact she had on all of us. A convocation of laughter and tears, of fondest reminiscences and those sights which will, for years to come constitute for some our bitterest memories.

Yes, she is gone. At 12:21 she breathed her last. She held on all day yesterday, refusing to even take morphine, waiting for Matthew and Emily to reach home.

We were together at the end, the four of us. Emily, Matthew, and me holding Mary and holding each other, and I never really realized until today what a family truly is. They have been like rocks in this time of their loss, so much stronger than I have been. In part, I realize, this is because they have lived the bulk of their adult lives with her death sentence looming over their heads. They have said their goodbyes intellectually and spiritually, the final departure lacking only the physical, spoken farewell.

Emily asked only one thing of her mother as we approached the end days, and that was for her not to die on her birthday. For the past week, Mary frequently asked what day it was, because she wished to comply with her wishes. And so she did, lasting two days past Emily's 32nd birthday.

Several of Emily's friends have visited, or written either notes or long, heartfelt letters to Mary, recounting what a tremendously positive influence she has been in their lives. One of them wrote, "Thank you for making us all better women."

She touched so many people in so many ways. One thing you cannot cheat is another person's heart, and this she never even tried. She thought the best of everyone, and tried to temper those less charitable impulses in me. She never took, only gave. She was depressed, to the best of my memory, exactly once in her life, and was mystified by that experience. I remember thinking, "Welcome to my world."

I don't know that I ever let her fully into that world. I'm not sure she ever would have really understood the maelstrom which is my consciousness. I don't regret it. I don't regret looking at her, back in college those decades back, and thinking, and saying to my friend Tim Jones, "I'm going to marry that girl."

I told her, too, on our first date, and for some reason, that failed to scare her away. So maybe she saw something too. Maybe she somehow ferreted out some inner quality that made her think it would perhaps be worthwhile for her to allow me to tag along with her in life.

Mary always thought the best of everyone, and if she didn't, then you were a particularly useless piece of human flotsam.

I remember once, when I lived in San Francisco, and was going through a particularly difficult period in my life, I made a new friend, Bob Houseman, let us call him, who rapidly became my best friend. What a wonderful man he was, a boundless personality, someone who lifted you up and made you shine.

When Mary came for a visit, I couldn't wait for them to meet. I couldn't wait to show off the friend in whose presence I reflected so brightly. I remember so vividly riding down Lincoln Boulevard on a brilliant sun-spanked day, in Bob's Fiat Spitfire convertible, cherry red, of course, with Mary in the passenger seat and me sprawled across the back, tooling alongside Golden Gate Park. It is a memory which remains indelibly imprinted on my mind.

I don't remember where we went next, or what we did, but it was a perfect day. Until he dropped us off, and I said to Mary, "Isn't Bob great?" And she said no. No, he wasn't great. She thought he was false. She thought he was dishonest. I was hurt by her lack of regard, by her blatant hostility. I questioned her judgment and thought she was wrong, wrong, wrong. Until just a matter of days later, when Bob proved how right she was. I don't even remember what he did, or what he said, but whatever he did was the kind of thing that friends didn't do to friends. It was the kind of betrayal that fundamentally dishonest people commit.

Bob had entered not just my life. He had become that person to so many of us, and none of us recognized he was a fundamentally dishonest person, except Mary. Mary, who never judged anyone, judged him, and found him wanting.

That's what I lost today. She left a Mary-sized hole in my soul that memories alone can never fill. She left two wonderful kids with a future bright and beautiful. She left a life she filled with beauty and grace. She left a circle of friends, a circle larger than she ever knew of people of who loved and valued her.

And she left me. The doctor gave her a year. She took six, and they were wonderful years together. I told her early in this journey if she was strong enough, she could help me get through this. She was. Strong enough for us both. I know life goes on, and so will I. But for now, I want just want to sit alone in the dark for a month or two, or maybe three. And then we'll see.

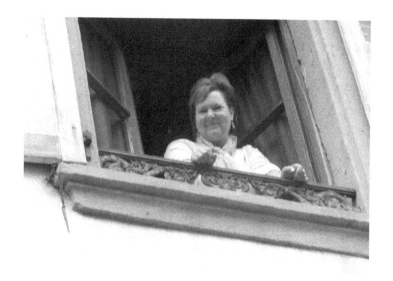

October 6, 2016
The Road is Long

With many a winding turn, that leads us to who knows where. It's been three months now, and this is what I'm reduced to, quoting the lyrics of sappy sixties-era pop ballads.

It has been a whirlwind of activity, life best spent in a haze of busyness. I bought a house, cut down trees, built a fence, went to California, harvested grapes, and went to funerals. Three funerals in four weeks; one, Larry's, two weeks after Mary's, in the same church with most of the same people in attendance. Then Bruce, his long fight against cancer undermined by an infection. Cancer is a vindictive bug. Five times it came at Bruce, and five times it failed, but like the intrepid spider in Robert the Bruce's hovel, it would not give up.

I thought, at Larry's funeral, that I wasn't really there, but rather reliving Mary's. I thought then it had cost me two weeks of recovery. But I was wrong. This isn't the kind of thing you can recover from on a schedule. You don't heal, as from a wound, or an injury. You don't start to get better once treatment begins. Rather than scar tissue forming, the more apt analogy is the phantom pain the amputee suffers in that foot or leg or arm, or in this case the heart, that has been surgically removed.

The unexpected thing as that with the passage of time it grows harder, not easier. I suppose in part it's because the burst of energy dissipates in time. One doesn't want to call it excitement, but in a way it is, especially when you're heading down a path you've never walked before. Everything is new, and you can spend your time learning a new language, solving puzzles you never knew existed, spending seemingly hours on the phone reciting strings of numbers, her birthday, the date of her death, "the last four of her social," (which is, incidentally, a phrase the repetition of which ought to be a felony), your phone number, your date of birth, etc, etc, etc.

In time, funeral arrangements finalized, guest housing secured, ceremony done, wake concluded, hugs exchanged, the last friend or sibling or offspring departed, and you settle down to an empty house.

Keep busy, they say. Good advice, that, as far as it goes. You can stay busy, and active, and it is good, but in the end, all you're trying to do is outrun the grief, and sooner or later, you have to pause to catch your breath, and it is there. Grief, you learn eventually, is a lot like cancer. It can afford to be patient, because it knows in time you will let down your guard and then it will strike.

Never turn down an invitation, they say. Maybe, though I have turned down some. Sometimes you need to be alone. You can be alone, I've always known, and not be lonely, but I've come to understand that you can be lonely when surrounded by friends. Sometimes, I wonder, is this becoming a habit? Here's something odd I've discovered. My entire life I've been perfectly comfortable dining out alone. I haven't felt strange, or lonely or anything other than content to sit at a table by myself, with maybe a book or magazine to amuse me between courses. Since Mary died, I've done it only rarely. It just doesn't feel right.

Yes, I've turned down invitations to join others. Not

always, but often. There remains a cautionary voice, warning me that if I don't say yes sometimes, in time, they will stop asking.

I've declined offers of food. I don't need someone to cook for me. In fact, preparing food has been a form of spiritual sustenance. I've developed the habit of walking the aisles of a grocery store, waiting for things to jump off the shelf, and deciding how to put them together. Sort of my own private Cooking Channel reality show.

I spoke with a recent widow who told me one of the hardest parts is the words of condolence. I get it. After three months it's still so fresh, those you see who haven't said it feel obligated to say they're sorry. Of course they do, it would be unnatural not to. But how are we, the grieving, supposed to respond? The reflexive response, the one best choked back and suppressed, is "What? Did you think I'd forgotten?" Unnecessary, of course. That's not what they meant, that's not what they meant at all.

So why does it keep getting harder? Because, I suppose, all those things that once reminded you of her still do, not with diminishing impact, but with a sort of cumulative weight. "No, she's not here," they seem to say. "She's not here, and she never will be."

With the exception of one book review, and the occasional Facebook post, I hadn't written a single word since Mary died. I was mystified by that development. Would I ever write again, I wondered? Would it be so bad if I didn't? Then, a couple of weeks ago, I started thinking "That would make a good story," or "Here's a nice turn of phrase." So maybe I'm starting to come out of it. I do know I woke up today and felt the need to file an update to the Cancer Blog.

Maybe that's a good thing, or maybe you're thinking, "Oh no. He's back."

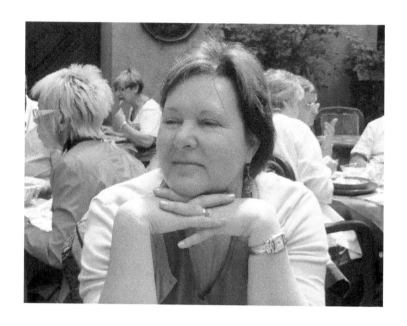